# How to Stop Cavities

## A Natural Approach to

## Prevention and Remineralization

# Judene Benoit, DDS

**Disclaimer**

This publication contains the opinions and ideas of the author and cannot be used as, or as a substitute for, diagnosis or treatment of any dental or medical concern. This publication does not provide a basis for action in any circumstance without seeking the diagnosis and advice of a qualified dentist, physician, or other licensed healthcare professional. The author expressly disclaims any responsibility for any liability, loss, or risk, personal or otherwise, which is incurred as a consequence, directly or indirectly, of the use and application of any of the contents of this book.

Cover design: Jay Dwyer
Edited by: Christine Pillman

ISBN 978-0-9939488-0-0

Printed in Canada

This book is dedicated to:

My Dad,

for teaching me what I know about dentistry, for without him this book could not be possible,

My Mom,

for believing in me even when I didn't,

Cara, my dog,

for bringing so much joy into my life,

&

Andre,

my husband and soul mate,

for making me the luckiest girl in the world

by being my man,

and for giving me the greatest gift in the world, your love.

# Table of Contents

# 1

# The Ah, Ha! Moment

"The caries [cavity] process is endemic and potentially both preventable and curable. The latter can be achieved by identifying and arresting or reversing the disease at an early stage."

*– National Institute of Health Consensus Statement*[1]

The crowd went wild, hooting and clapping. The roar of the crowd continued while I scrubbed away at a crusty stain on my kitchen counter. Oh, good, it came off, I thought to myself. The cheering finally started to subside, and the speaker began talking again. I stopped scrubbing the counter and turned my attention to the iPad where a video of a famous health and wellness expert was playing on YouTube. "I must have missed something. Why is the audience cheering so much?" I said aloud. I dragged the play bar back and listened again. The speaker said he healed one of his teeth and didn't need to get a filling done. Then the crowd went wild. Like really wild. I paused the video, squinted my eyes with a puzzled look on my face. I was confused. Why was the crowd so incredibly excited over a healed tooth? Don't get me wrong, I thought a healed tooth was exciting, but it was in the same category as a healed skin wound to me. Exciting yes, but not newsworthy. See, every day at work I would see a ton of healed teeth.

And just then a big "ah, ha!" moment came over me, dirty dish scrubber in one hand and iPad in the other. "Holy crow! There are people who don't realize teeth can heal!"

Over the next few weeks, I decided to test out this new theory in my dental office. Every time I'd see a healed tooth, I would hand the person a mirror and point to the spots on their teeth. "Did you know that a cavity started here a while ago but you healed it up?" I would ask. The responses were quite varied, but the general theme was shock. Most people would say something along the lines of, "Really? I didn't know cavities could heal."

Every dentist knows that cavities can heal, although the word "healed" is generally not used to describe the phenomenon. "Remineralization" and "arrested decay" are the proper dental terms used to refer to the concept of healing.[2] In fact, all of the following terms can be used either formally or informally to confer the same meaning:

-Preventing cavities
-Healthy teeth
-Reversed cavity
-Reversed decay
-Healed cavity
-Hardened teeth
-Hardened cavity
-Arrested decay
-Stopped cavity

Throughout this book I use all these terms interchangeably.


## Healing & Cavities

Healing a tooth or cavity does not mean that the missing tooth structure will grow back. Let's pretend someone accidentally cuts their fingertip off. When the finger heals, there is a solid layer of skin formed at the site of the injury that is comparable to the rest of the skin on the finger. The healed finger no longer has a risk of infection spreading, and is functioning in a rather normal state that doesn't require surgical intervention, unless for cosmetic or other reasons to replace the missing fingertip. Part of the healing process for the finger however, did not involve the fingertip growing back.

This is similar to what happens when a cavity is healed or arrested or remineralized – remember they mean the same thing. The site of the cavity becomes hard and has a composition comparable to the rest of the tooth. There is no longer risk of the cavity spreading or growing, and the tooth functions in a normal state that doesn't require surgical intervention, unless for cosmetic or other reasons to replace the missing tooth structure with a filling or some other restoration.[3] And just like the finger, part of the healing process for the tooth and cavity does not involve the piece of missing tooth growing back.

To reiterate, the word, "healed" in reference to a tooth or cavity does not suggest that a tooth or part of a tooth will grow back. Fingertips don't grow back, but the skin heals; teeth don't grow back, but the tooth surface heals.[4]

This book is based on two main concepts:

1. Remineralization, (or prevention, healing, reversing, arresting or however one wishes to say it,) of both teeth and cavities is possible. Dentists are taught this in dental school, and

remineralization is often a major focus in the modern dental office.

2. *Natural* remineralization, (or prevention, healing, reversing, arresting) of cavities is possible. Although there are some other strategies used, most remineralization strategies today are focused on fluoride and oral-hygiene techniques. There are, however, many additional tools that can be employed that will potentiate whichever current methods of remineralization you are utilizing. Due to an increased movement from the general public towards more natural approaches to dentistry, as well as my own personal interest in health and wellness, these additional aspects I discuss are based on natural strategies. The number one reason I promote natural approaches to remineralization is the added benefits of positively affecting overall health as well as oral health.[5]

In addition to making recommendations based on present and past published research studies, as well as what I was taught in dental school, I also use the knowledge of my own experiences – what I have seen with my own two eyes, both clinically and personally. Not only is it possible to prevent and remineralize cavities, but it is possible to do so naturally!

Prevention and remineralization of cavities is a reality. Whether you have heard of remineralization or not, and whether you know what remineralization of teeth means or not, it doesn't matter. It's happening in your mouth anyway.[6] Or at least trying to. Our body is designed to prevent and heal cavities. All we have to do is set our body up for success and let it do its thing.[7] There is no wrong way to remineralize your teeth – only many, many right ways. Indeed, there are people either in the past or present who have successfully healed cavities in wildly different ways than the next person. The key is that it is possible, and to find what works best for you.

## Why Bother to Prevent and Remineralize Cavities?

I was attending a dental lecture about (synthetic) remineralizing techniques. The dentist lecturing discussed many different techniques for several hours. At the end of the lecture, a dentist in the audience raised his hand and said something of the following, "Remineralization sounds great, but the reality is that it is so much work and most of my patients tell me that having a filling is no longer a big deal. Why would they care to do anything but just get a filling for a cavity?"

Absolutely, remineralizing your teeth and cavities requires much more work and effort than having a filling done. And *naturally* remineralizing your teeth and cavities requires even *more* work and effort.

Quite often, having fillings and other restorative dental work completed is the best answer for some people. Indeed, modern dentistry has made it possible to have quality restorative treatments completed in a relaxed and even enjoyable manner. There is certainly nothing wrong with having fillings and restorative work completed, if that is what you want and/or that is the best course of action for you and your family. However, for some people, including myself, natural (or synthetically-based) prevention and remineralization is preferred over restorative treatments. The following is a list of reasons why one might consider the extra effort of natural prevention and remineralization to be worthwhile.

1. Dental restorations do not last forever. While some materials last for many years and in some individuals, their lifetime, this is the exception as opposed to the norm.[8]

2. All fillings and restorations are susceptible to recurrent decay, which is a new cavity formed around an existing restoration. Existing fillings and restorations will last longer and be less susceptible to recurrent decay and to breakage when remineralization strategies are utilized.[9,10,11] I often hear people say they can't get any more cavities because all their teeth are already filled. This is not true. Not only can cavities develop on a different part of a tooth that already has a filling, but a cavity can develop right on an existing filling (recurrent decay). Some fillings last longer, much longer, than others, and having a tooth remineralized as opposed to

demineralized will certainly favor a longer lasting restoration.[12,13]

3. Any time the tooth is drilled, there is the potential for irritation and damage to the nerve. This could result in sensitivity, either temporary or long-term, nerve death and infection requiring a root canal or extraction.[14,15]

4. Many dental materials have the potential to release cytotoxic components, the levels of which have been determined to be safe.[16] For example, amalgam restorations are known to release mercury, however the amount of mercury released is considered to be safe. Composite fillings, as well as bonds or "glue" for porcelain restorations are known to release bisphenol A (BPA), an endocrine disruptor, but the amount released is considered to be safe.[17,18,19]

5. Fillings and other restorative treatments do not address the underlying cause(s) of why a cavity developed in the first place. Without dealing with the underlying cause(s), one is at very high risk of having another cavity in the future. [20]

## Acute vs Chronic Treatments

Modern dentistry and dental materials are remarkably advanced, and, of course, very useful. For example, accidents involving teeth can so negatively affect someone's life, and thankfully dentists and dental technologies are able to help. Even the most severe dental deformities can be repaired and the person can be given their life back. However, in cases of chronic dental disease, it is ideal to move away from a situation of chronic disease and chronic treatments to one of health, where restorations are limited.

Nothing beats our own natural teeth. Today we are fortunate to have a large array of great dental materials, but no dental material can compete with a healthy and strong tooth.

## To Restore or Not to Restore

Of course it sounds so wonderful to remineralize a cavity and not need a filling, but there are potentially some serious risks involved.

As a dentist, I find the subject of stopping cavities to be a delicate balance between giving people the positive hope of a cavity-free mouth and not giving them the false hope of a cavity-free mouth. I want people to know that it is indeed possible to have a cavity-free mouth; that it is possible to remineralize teeth and cavities, and to do it naturally. However I also want people to know that it may not be possible for everyone, for one reason or another. I have seen many times people successfully arrest their cavities. I have also seen many people who have been unsuccessful in arresting their cavities, and end up having fillings done, developing new cavities, needing a root canal or teeth extracted. I have seen people cry tears of joy and cry out of frustration and sadness.

One thing I can say for sure is that I recommend everyone to remineralize their teeth as a preventive measure. In other words, to remineralize their teeth before a cavity forms.

**Remineralize _Teeth_ = Prevention of cavities**

**Remineralize _Cavity_ = Cavity already formed, but no restorative treatment necessary**

Remineralizing your _teeth_ will always prove to be beneficial, resulting in stronger teeth that are more resistant to decay. However, taking remineralizing even further, in an attempt to remineralize an existing cavity to avoid getting a filling, is potentially a much more risky endeavor that may or may not be best for an individual. Focusing on the general remineralization of teeth (aka prevention) is something for everyone, and focusing on remineralizing an existing cavity should be made on an individual basis, with supervision by a dentist. Information about risks and benefits is imperative to help someone make the best choice for themselves and their family.

Risks versus Benefits:

**Risks of naturally remineralizing teeth**

**= None! (this is prevention of cavities)**

**Risks of naturally or synthetically attempting to reminer-
alize an existing cavity**

**= Small to huge potential problems**

The risk of not having a restoration done and instead working to remineralize a cavity always poses the possibility that the cavity might not remineralize or arrest. If the cavity does not remineralize, it will continue to progress and this is never good. If an active, progressing cavity is left, there will always be problems, quite often big problems. The following is a list of potential problems that could occur either separately or jointly at once:

· The tooth could break

· The tooth could break so much that it is no longer restorable

· The tooth could become infected

· The tooth could become mildly to unbearably painful

· The tooth could need a root canal or extraction

All of the above could happen while on vacation far away from any emergency care!

## Systemic Benefits from Naturally Remineralizing

My passion for systemic or overall health improvements is one of the main reasons why I promote natural prevention and remineralization. It is very nice to see how happy someone is when told they have no cavities or that their cavity is remineralized after using synthetic approaches. However, I feel tremendous amounts of joy to hear the stories of overall health benefits that go along with using natural approaches. Children once diagnosed with failure to thrive who are now healthy, cleared up allergies and acne, improved energy, weight normalization, improved school performance, better sleep and disappeared rashes – these and others are health benefits experienced by people who take a natural approach to their normal prevention techniques. I didn't even know they had these problems, and sometimes neither did they until the problems went away. By improving one's oral health naturally, systemic health will inadvertently benefit as well. What's good for the goose is good for the gander, and what's good for the teeth is good for the body!

Is it more work and more challenging to use natural approaches to improve oral health? Absolutely. But I personally think it is well worth it. I wish I could, but I cannot say that you will be able to remineralize a cavity. All I can say is that remineralizing your teeth so that you prevent getting a cavity in the first place is by far the most ideal situation.

**Always remember: choosing not to have fillings done can be a risky endeavor. The best route is to remineralize your teeth before any cavities develop.**

# 2

# Cavities 101

"Unfortunately no dental material can completely replace real tooth structure. This is why prevention is so important. With proper care from you and your dentist – it is achievable to maintain oral health throughout a lifetime."

*– Canadian Dental Association website* [1]

N ow that you know the risks of attempting to remineralize a cavity, which can involve significant
risk, the following is information about remineralizing teeth and cavities so you can make an informed decision
about what is best for yourself and your family.

## What is a Cavity?

The current definition of a cavity is that it is the removal of
minerals by bacterial acids. It is an infection from bacteria,
which produce acid that removes minerals/tooth structure
from the tooth, and the removal of minerals leads to a hole –
a cavity.[2] Removal of minerals can be called demineralization,
dissolution or destruction of tooth.

**Bacteria →Acid**

**→Removal of Minerals or Tooth Structure**

**→Hole / Cavity**

Even though I will continue to use the term "cavity"
throughout this book, I want you to be aware that the proper
dental term for cavity is "caries." Often a cavity is referred to
as a "lesion." For example, a carious lesion is a cavity.

Very important point:

**Cavities are either active or arrested.[3]**

If a cavity is active, it is progressing or growing larger. An active cavity means continual demineralization, dissolution of minerals and destruction of tooth is occurring.

If a cavity is arrested, the cavity was active at some point, but has stopped progressing. There was demineralization in the past, but the cavity has since been remineralized. A cavity that is arrested is what some people call a healed cavity, or a reversed cavity. An arrested cavity usually does not require a filling, unless for cosmetic or some other desire.[4]

Most people consider cavities to be bad, or at least an unpleasant diagnosis. Active cavities are indeed bad, while arrested cavities are actually a really great diagnosis. Even though cavities can be either active or arrested, usually when one speaks of a cavity, they are referring to an active cavity. I would assume that if a dentist or dental professional is talking about a cavity, they are speaking of the active and progressing form. In this book, when the word cavity is used, I am referring to an active cavity. I will specify the inactive form of a cavity by calling it arrested, stopped, remineralized, healed or some similar term.

**Cavity = Arrested or Active**

**Cavity = Not Necessarily Bad**

**Active Cavity = Bad/Unpleasant Diagnosis**

**Arrested Cavity = Great Diagnosis**

An arrested cavity is not at any greater risk of becoming an active cavity again. Just because it was once active, that does not mean it is more likely to become active again. An arrested cavity either has the same risk of developing a cavity as the rest of the teeth or it has a lower risk of developing a cavity in the future. This is because during the process of remineralization, the tooth creates an even denser layer of minerals than the surrounding areas, as a form of protection.[5]

I like to compare arrested decay to a button on a shirt. Sometimes when I buy a shirt, a button comes loose very quickly. After I get out a needle and thread and stitch the button back on or reinforce it before it falls off, the button is very secure and won't fall off or come loose ever again, even though some of the other buttons may come loose and need to be restitched. The restitched buttons are much stronger than when the shirt was originally purchased, and this is a similar occurrence for arrested decay. Many people are quite concerned that arrested decay is more susceptible to a cavity in the future, but just like the reinforced buttons on a shirt, this is simply not the case.

## What is Remineralization?

Remineralization is a fancy-sounding word that means putting minerals back into the tooth. Demineralization is the opposite, and is the removal of minerals from the tooth. Enough removal of minerals, or demineralization, will lead to a hole in the tooth, known as a cavity.[6]

Healing a cavity may sound very complicated and newfangled, but it really is a normal process that thankfully happens all the time.[7] Without remineralization, none of us would have any teeth left, since demineralization and the loss of minerals happens so frequently with foods and drinks, and even while simply sitting at rest. Just like our skin sloughs off and is replaced seamlessly, so too are minerals lost from our teeth. We don't even know it's happening, but the minerals are replaced quickly and effectively so our teeth are strong, and we can happily chomp down the food during our next meal. For all those children and adults who have had a cavity or cavities, something has gone awry with the normal functioning abilities of the body, mouth and saliva, resulting in a cavity.[8]

A cavity results when the demineralization exceeds the remineralization. Even though the body is still most certainly remineralizing the rest of the teeth, in one particular area the demineralization has gotten ahead of the remineralization, resulting in the diagnosis of a cavity.[9]

**Demineralization > Remineralization = Active Cavity**

**Remineralization ≥ Demineralization = No Cavity or Arrested Cavity**

The key to naturally (or synthetically) healing your teeth is to slow down the process of demineralization and speed up the remineralization. Once we have a hole in our tooth, we cannot fill the hole in with more visible tooth structure, but we can make the hole lining more dense with minerals, resulting in a hardened cavity that will no longer progress.[10,11]

When remineralization or the deposition of missing minerals from a tooth occurs at a very early stage with only a small amount of minerals, this is what people call prevention of cavities. When you go to the dentist no cavities are found.

**Remineralization $\geq$ Tiny Area of Demineralization**

**= Prevention of Cavities**

When the process of remineralization occurs after a large amount of minerals were lost, this is known as an arrested cavity or arrested decay.

**Remineralization $\geq$ Enough Demineralization to be Seen Either with X-rays or the Eye**

**= Arrested Decay**

Thus, the process of both prevention of cavities and healing of cavities is the same. Remineralization is what this process is usually called. Remineralization is good, demineralization is bad.

# A Little Anatomy

The crown is the part of the tooth above the gums, and is the part that is visible and with which we chew. The outer layer of the crown is called enamel, which is on average 1.2 mm thick, but varies depending on location as well as by how much has been worn away. Enamel is the hardest substance found in the body – harder than bone![12] The crown of the tooth is not to be confused with a crown that is a restoration done by a dentist, which covers the crown of the tooth.

Underneath enamel is dentin. Dentin is much more porous than enamel. In fact, microscopically the structure of dentin is a series of many tiny tubes called tubules. These tiny tubes extend from the pulp to the enamel.[13]

The very middle of the insides of a tooth is the pulp. The pulp contains blood and lymph vessels, as well as nerves that are connected to blood and lymph vessels and nerves in the rest of the body.[14]

The root is the part of the tooth that we don't see – it is inside the bone and surrounded by gums, or gingiva. The root surface is not made of enamel, it is made of something called cementum. Cementum is very thin and is also more porous than enamel. Dentin in underneath the thin layer of cementum. Dentin comprises most of both the root and the crown of a tooth, and therefore makes up the majority of a tooth.[15]

# Hydroxyapatite

When minerals are discussed as being removed or deposited into enamel and the tooth, the specific molecule involved is called hydroxyapatite. Hydroxyapatite is made up of minerals, and when minerals are said to be lost or replaced, it is the hydroxyapatite minerals that this is in reference to.

The chemical composition of hydroxyapatite is:

$Ca_{10}(PO_4)_6(OH)_2$.

Ca = Calcium

$PO_4$ = Phosphate

OH = Hydroxyl

Enamel is composed of hydroxyapatite, and so is dentin. (Remember enamel is composed of densely packed hydroxyapatite, whereas dentin has tubes within it, making it much more porous.)

# Odontoblasts

The odontoblast is a funny-sounding name but is an incredibly important cell within teeth. In fact, the odontoblast is my favorite part of teeth! Odontoblasts are part of both dentin and pulp tissues because their cell bodies reside in the pulp, but their long, slender cytoplasmic cell processes (Tomes fibers) extend into the dentin tubes. It is as if the odontoblasts sit in the pulp and have long skinny arms that reach out into dentin. Odontoblasts make teeth alive! I know that it sounds weird to think that teeth are alive, but because odontoblasts are capable of reacting to physiologic and pathologic stimuli, dentin is considered to be a living tissue.[16]

Odontoblasts are responsible for making dentin. Dentin that is made when the tooth is first formed is called primary dentin.[17] Odontoblasts also make dentin throughout the life of the tooth in response to stimuli as an effort to protect the tooth from harm, such as cavities or drilling.[18] This protective dentin can be referred to as secondary or reparative dentin.[19,20] For example, in response to a slowly moving cavity, odontoblasts will produce more dentin in an effort to slow the cavity even more and to protect the pulp from infection. The protective or reparative dentin is said to be remineralized, and the new, more dense dentin cells are also called eburnated or 'sclerotic dentin.'[21]

Odontoblasts are sort of like brick layers working on a house. Except instead of the brick layers finishing their job and leaving, these brick layers stay forever at the house constantly repairing the brick walls. When an insect tries to make a home in between the brick, the brick layers quickly lay down more brick or mortar to patch it up. The house does not get bigger, but damage is repaired. Remember, even though new dentin can be continually produced, this does not mean the dentin will get bigger and the tooth can grow back – indeed that definitely does not happen! Dentin is not like your hair or fingernails that continue growing in size even when they are cut. Dentin is more like your skin cells that are replaced when sloughed off – new cells are made, but your skin does not increase in size. If an injury results in a finger being severed, the skin produces new skin to heal the area, but does not grow the finger back.

Secondary and reparative dentin that is made to protect the tooth, (called sclerotic and eburnated dentin), is denser than normal dentin, and behaves more like enamel.[22] This more mineralized and dense dentin is more resistant to decay than normal dentin, and is so dense that it can even make bonding a filling to the area more difficult.[23] Another way to think about it is to imagine a piece of Swiss cheese with lots of holes in it. Remineralizing dentin with new reparative dentin is like filling in the holes in the piece of cheese. The cheese becomes denser and less porous, but does not increase in size.

Odontoblasts do not extend into enamel, and as such, additional enamel can't be made again after tooth development.

## Dentin Remineralization

In dental school, one of my favorite instructors was a dentist who worked at his office four days a week and helped out at the dental school on Fridays. He was one of my favorites because he was just a really great person. He was easy to talk to, was always positive and had a wealth of great information and tips to teach and advise the students. He was probably in his fifties, if I had to guess. He clearly had a lot of experience and was also up to date on modern practices. One day we were being taught about dentin remineralization and some dental procedures that rely on successful dentin remineralization – direct and indirect pulp capping and overdentures. At the end of the lecture, which was given by another dentist, my favorite dental instructor, who happened to be standing next to me, turned to me and said, "That doesn't work." "Really?" I asked, shocked. "It always fails," he said politely, while shaking his head. "Don't bother, you'll waste your time." "Hmm, okay thanks," I said, a little disappointed.

Since that discussion, I have spoken with many dentists who feel the same way as my favorite dental instructor. They feel that even though the theory of dentin remineralization exists, the reality of it is nonexistent.

I understand why dentin cavities have developed the reputation of being impossible to remineralize. I won't deny that yes, probably for some people, dentin remineralization is not a reality. For those people, dentin remineralization will simply remain a great theory, as opposed to reality. However, for some people, with the necessary conditions in place, the theory of dentin remineralization is a reality.

Dentin remineralization is a reality, however it is much more difficult to achieve than enamel remineralization.[24,25,26] Think of your skin as enamel, and the soft tissue underneath your thick skin as dentin. If you get a cut in your skin, it is not very deep, and it's within the thick, tough outer layer. The wound will likely heal without much difficultly. If, however, you get a deep cut that goes through to the soft tissue under your skin, you would likely require some significant healing time or even stitches. It certainly does not heal as easily as the shallow cut. A cavity extending into dentin is like a deep wound. While healing is possible, it is certainly much more difficult for the body to accomplish.[27] Sometimes major complications or problems can arise from a lack of dentin healing, and sometimes surgical intervention is the best route of action.

## Remineralization Likeliness

Cavities vary significantly in their likeliness to remineralize, depending on their size and location on the tooth. Of course, no cavity or tooth will ever remineralize if the necessary conditions to do so are not met. But even when necessary techniques are utilized and the conditions are in favor of remineralization, some cavities are easier to remineralize than others. Some are so challenging they might never remineralize. (These necessary conditions will be covered in subsequent chapters.)

### Size of the Cavity

Cavities that are located in the enamel only are very small, since enamel is only 1.2 mm or less in thickness. These cavities, called incipient cavities, are significantly easier to remineralize than cavities extending beyond enamel into dentin. A larger cavity means a larger loss of minerals, and a smaller cavity has fewer minerals missing. Since stopping a cavity involves replacing the lost minerals, it makes sense then that the fewer minerals needed to be replaced, the easier and quicker and more likely it will happen.

Let's pretend you are doing a thousand-piece puzzle and accidentally drop some puzzle pieces. If you dropped one puzzle piece on the floor, it would be much more likely that you will find it and finish the puzzle. But if you dropped 999 puzzle pieces on the floor, finding them all becomes a huge undertaking. It will take more effort, more time and you may not even be able to find them all. This is the same for replacing lost minerals from a tooth or cavity in order to remineralize it. The more minerals that have been lost, the more effort and time will be necessary to do so, and some people may not ever be able to completely remineralize their teeth and cavities.

## Location of the Cavity

Our saliva is designed to remineralize our teeth and cavities; in fact, remineralization is one of its main functions.[28,29] Provided we set up the conditions necessary for successful remineralization, our saliva will be able to do its job. Any part of the tooth that is easily accessed by saliva will therefore be the easiest and quickest to remineralize, while those parts hidden from saliva will pose the most difficultly.[30]

## Smooth Surfaces

The easiest cavities to remineralize (assuming necessary conditions are met) are those on smooth surfaces. Smooth surfaces on a tooth are the cheek-side and tongue-side of the tooth; the surfaces touching the lips and cheeks, called facial and labial surfaces and the surfaces touching or facing the tongue, called lingual surfaces. The smooth surfaces are the flat parts of the teeth that you can touch and see. Cavities located on these surfaces are easily accessed by saliva and are smooth with little impedance to remineralization.

## Biting Surface

A very common spot for cavities to occur is on the biting surface, called the occlusal surface. Thankfully, this is a spot that the saliva does have access to, and is a realistic location to remineralize. However, because the deep grooves on teeth provide a good hiding spot for bacteria, these cavities are more challenging to remineralize than smooth surface cavities, but generally saliva is still able to access the grooves.

# Interproximal Surfaces

Interproximal or proximal surfaces are the surfaces that touch other teeth. This is the part of the tooth that one flosses. Even though these parts of the tooth are smooth surfaces, cavities in between teeth definitely do not behave as smooth surface cavities because of the very limited access to saliva. Cavities that are located on interproximal surfaces are among the most challenging to remineralize and are also the most challenging to monitor and assess because they are not visible to the naked eye or easily accessed.

Many times a cavity forms like a tunnel or a triangle with the pointy end into the dentin. This gives the inside portion of the cavity very limited access to saliva. Imagine now that the tunnel or triangle cavity is located in between teeth. The deepest part of the cavity already has limited access but when it resides in between teeth, there is essentially no access to saliva. With no access to saliva, which contains the minerals necessary to do the remineralizing, remineralization will not occur. Let's pretend that remineralization is comparable to stomping on dirt to harden the surface. If the surface you want to stomp on is inside a rabbit hole, you aren't going to be able to stomp on it. Just like if the dentin that needs to be remineralized is deep within a tunnel cavity, especially if it is in between teeth, remineralization will not occur.

Now let's compare the tunnel cavity deep within dentin to dentin remineralization that does often occur – such as when a dentist exposes dentin for the purpose of an overdenture. Overdentures involve wearing a denture over top of drilled down teeth (or implants) in order to preserve bone structure.[31] Today using natural drilled down teeth is not done as much because implants are usually used instead. However, the process involves the dentist drilling off the whole crown, or the visible part of the tooth, doing a root canal and continually focusing on remineralization of the now exposed dentin so that a cavity does not develop. Although certainly sometimes these teeth do get cavities, often it is a successful treatment and dentin remineralization is achieved. But the situation is drastically different than a tunnel cavity extending into dentin hidden from saliva. The overdenture tooth has complete access to saliva, there are no hidden areas for a cavity to hide from saliva, and therefore dentin remineralization is a reality. This would be like stomping on soil that is in a garden. Access is easy and stomping on the soil will likely happen. The only time I usually recommend considering an attempt to remineralize dentin (which again, is not for everyone) is when the dentin has significant exposure to the saliva.

## Structural Changes

Sometimes enamel or tooth structure will flake away from a cavity, whether it is arrested or active. This could be the sign of a problem and progressing cavity, indicating that further destruction of the tooth is continuing to occur. If the cavity is already arrested, flaking away tooth structure does not usually pose a problem. Flaking away tooth structure means that at some point the area was weakened, or 'undermined,' in dental terminology. Quite often, an undermined area of the tooth will not actually flake away at the moment it becomes undermined or weakened. It may flake away at a much later time, even after the cavity or tooth has remineralized.

This may be difficult to understand because an arrested cavity is strong and sometimes even stronger than the surrounding tooth, so it might seem like the tooth should not be crumbling away after being arrested. Or one might think it is a sign that the cavity is not arrested and is in fact active.

Certainly most of the time, crumbling and flaking teeth do occur in the presence of active cavities. I do not want to falsely lead one to believe that a breaking tooth is a good thing. I just want to make it clear that it is not always a sign of active decay. An arrested cavity can have structural changes that do not necessarily mean the cavity is active again.

If the cavity is active and slowly progressing, flaking away tooth structure could actually make the cavity easier to remineralize, due to the increased exposure to saliva. Remember dentin cavities must have exposure to saliva in order to remineralize, and this exposure will occur either through tooth shape and/or chipping away of the covering enamel.[32]

Imagine the dirt deep within a rabbit hole that you are trying to access. All of a sudden, the grass and soil covering the hole has been removed. Now you can stomp on the dirt.

## Recurrent Decay

Recurrent decay is a cavity that forms around an existing restoration. Recurrent decay is extremely challenging to remineralize. Sometimes there is no access to saliva, and sometimes the decay is due to an issue with the restoration, such as breakdown of adhesives or slight shrinkage of the filling.

### Review

So let's review: a cavity in the enamel that is located on the cheek-side or tongue-side of a tooth will be easiest to remineralize, provided the necessary conditions are met, of course. A cavity extending into the dentin in between teeth or under a filling will be the most challenging to remineralize, and everything else falls somewhere in between.

**No cavity will remineralize, even if it is tiny in the easiest location, if the necessary conditions are not met!**

# Remineralization Likeliness Chart

The Remineralization Likeliness Chart* gives you an idea of the chances of having successful remineralization, if you have the necessary conditions in order to do so. Remember, no cavity will remineralize, even if it is most likely to, without the necessary conditions in place, which are covered in subsequent chapters. Ask your dentist about the size and surfaces of your cavity, and discuss your desires to attempt remineralization. Your dentist will know how likely your cavity is to remineralize. Please note that this guide is mostly based on my opinion only, and if your dentist recommends something different, you should follow your dentist's advice. I also recommend writing down what your dentist and hygienist say during your appointment because these dental terms are easy to forget. The size of a cavity extending into the dentin is usually determined by looking at X-rays, although visual inspection is sometimes possible, depending on the location. For example, a cavity is easier to see on the biting surface. Cavity detection devices that use methods other than radiation may also be used to indicate cavity size.

*Based on author's opinion with select references.[33,34,35]

Note: A cavity on a surface that normally would be touching another tooth (interproximal) but the other tooth is missing is counted as a cheek-side/tongue-side surface instead.

## Size Point(s):

Within Enamel (incipient) = 1

Into Dentin – Slightly = 4

Into Dentin - Moderately = 6

Into Dentin - Extensively = 7

Into Dentin and Enamel Chipped Away = minus 2

Into Dentin and Enamel Covering = 0

Recurrent Decay but Just Superficial Staining = minus 2

## Location Point(s):

Biting Surface of Molar/Premolar (Occlusal) = 2

Biting Surface of Front Teeth (Incisal) = 1

Cheek-Side (Facial/Buccal/Vestibular) = 1

Tongue-Side (Lingual) = 1

Between Teeth (Interproximal) = 4

Recurrent Decay (Touching an Existing Filling) = 5

Root Surface (Cementum) = 2

Developing Tooth = add 2

Add the Size Points & the
Location Points together:

**Easiest:** 2

**Challenging:** 3-6

**Highly Unlikely:** 7 and up

## Easiest Category

Remineralizing, or attempting to remineralize cavities that score in the easiest category is a great place to start for much of the population. Many people are able to remineralize these types of cavities with little (or even no noticeable) lifestyle changes. The risk of attempting to remineralize these cavities is very small, assuming regular visits to a dental office to make sure the cavity does not grow large, should remineralization not occur. Due to the small size of these cavities, a little cavity growth (if remineralization doesn't happen) between dental appointments would be highly unlikely to cause major dental problems.

## Challenging Category

Attempting to remineralize a cavity in the challenging category poses greater risk. The only people who should attempt to remineralize these cavities are those who are highly motivated to make some significant changes in their health and lifestyle, and are prepared to accept the risks and consequences if the cavity does not remineralize. Attempting to remineralize the challenging category of cavities is not for everyone.

Some people do not want to accept the risks if the cavity does not remineralize and grows. Some people might find themselves choosing to have a restoration done because it is not the best time in their life to attempt to remineralize a cavity. For example, someone who is interested in making lifestyle changes in the future but is too busy at the moment, would be best to have the cavity restored, and focus on remineralizing their teeth to prevent future cavities. For someone who is working very hard to ensure the necessary conditions for remineralization, even though challenging, remineralizing cavities in this category is a doable and realistic endeavor for someone to undertake.

## Highly Unlikely

I do not recommend attempting to remineralize any cavity which falls under the highly unlikely category. These cavities are so incredibly challenging to remineralize, and nearly always unsuccessful. I am not one to call anything impossible, but I encourage you to think of these cavities as impossible to remineralize.[36] With unsuccessful remineralization of these cavities, which will happen, the risks of losing the tooth, getting an infection or abscess or some other serious dental harm is extremely high. It is best to catch a cavity before it reaches this point, which is why it is a good idea to be seen regularly at a dental office. I have seen people refuse to have treatment completed for a cavity in the highly unlikely category. Despite my recommendation to have the cavities filled, these people refused (which is okay – it is their body), and told me they would be happier to have the tooth extracted than restored. Perhaps the cavity was on their wisdom tooth and they figured they wouldn't miss the tooth, or perhaps they just have some unique ideas that I cannot relate to, but of course they are entitled to. Most often these teeth do end up being extracted, breaking off or needing a root canal. Waiting for a cavity to be in this category is not ideal. Even if the cavity is restored at this point, the disadvantages of restorations are magnified when the restoration is large (such as risk of future abscess, breakage, long-term sensitivity...) Ideally, cavities would be diagnosed by routine dental care, and either be remineralized or restored before the cavity reaches this stage.

# Questions of Time

## Speed of Cavity Progression

How Fast Do Cavities Grow?

Cavities progress at different speeds ranging from quickly to slowly. This speed varies between individuals and even within an individual during different times of their life. Slow-growing cavities are far more likely to remineralize. With slow-growing cavities, the production of highly dense reparative dentin occurs as an effort to stop the cavity, regardless of whether the cavity is within the dentin or still just in the enamel. The quicker the progression of the cavity, the less likely the odontoblasts will be able to respond and make protective or reparative dentin.[37] Think of a car that loses its breaks and is heading toward a storefront filled with people. Imagine the car is traveling at a snail's pace. Someone in the store would notice it and yell out a warning, and the storefront would be cleared. There may have been time to call 911 before the car hit the window. Traveling at such a slow speed, the car would barely do any damage to the storefront, maybe not even breaking the glass. This is like a slowly progressing cavity. The tooth has time to defend itself and not much damage occurs. Now picture a car traveling at a high speed with no brakes toward a window. No one has time to see it and it smashes through the glass. Lots of damage occurs and people may have even been injured. This is like a rapidly progressing cavity. There is no time for the tooth to properly protect itself with new dense dentin, and the damage is extensive.

Cavity progression is a continuum, with extremes at both ends and everything in between. A very rapidly progressing cavity would be one that grows into dentin between routine dental appointments. A very slowly progressing cavity would be one that a dentist is observing for years and years. (A very slowly progressing cavity could easily be confused with arrested decay.) Most people have cavities somewhere in between these extremes.

Studies have shown that when risk factors are high, a cavity can develop in as little as three weeks.[38] An average amount of time for a cavity to appear clinically is around eighteen months plus or minus six months.[39] Cavity progression is slower in healthy individuals and more rapid in individuals with compromised health.[40]

If you or your child has rapidly progressing decay, I always recommend having a restoration completed instead of attempting to remineralize the cavity. Of course, focusing on remineralizing the rest of your teeth to prevent cavities is very important, and is a good aspect to focus on, instead of focusing on the cavity. I think that having a goal of reducing the speed of your cavity progression is where you should start. It would be almost, if not completely, impossible to go from having an extremely rapidly progressing cavity to one that is completely arrested. A more realistic goal is to focus on changing the speed of your cavities from rapidly progressing to slowly progressing. Then, in the future, another goal can be to take slowly progressing cavities to the point of remineralization and then to prevention. For example, a friend of mine had rapidly progressing cavities. In between routine dental appointments, she would develop cavities so large that they extended into the pulp and she would need root canals. This happened to her three times, then she decided to make some major changes in her diet and lifestyle. She developed two more medium-sized cavities and had them restored. This was a great accomplishment, because she was able to slow the speed of her cavity growth so that she had medium-sized cavities, as opposed to huge cavities between appointments. Once she was able to slow down the speed of her cavities, her next goal was to prevent new cavity development and remineralize tiny cavities. She has been successfully cavity free for years now. Had she decided to attempt to remineralize her cavities without first slowing down the speed of cavity growth, she would surely have a mouth full of root canals and/or missing teeth.

The steps to reducing the speed of cavity progression are exactly the same as the steps involved with cavity prevention and remineralization. (Remember a cavity that has slowed down so much that it has stopped progression is actually an arrested or remineralized or healed cavity.) Even though the steps are the same, the goals are much more realistic and much less risky. Taking several stages to achieve your overall goal of no new cavities will take more time, but will also be more likely to occur successfully.

**Rapidly Progressing Cavity → Completely Remineralized**

**= Not Likely and Very Risky**

Better Approach:

Rapidly Progressing Cavity: Have Restored

→ Slowly Progressing Cavity: Have Restored

→ Very Slowly Progressing Cavity: Remineralized

→ No New Cavities

## How Long Does it Take to Arrest & Remineralize a Cavity?

The answer to this question is that is varies drastically. Indeed, some people will never arrest their cavities, while others will do so very quickly. It depends on the size and the location of the cavity, as well as the internal and environmental factors relating to the tooth and individual. Generally speaking, remineralization is a very quick process. When the necessary factors are in place, the natural process of remineralization rapidly produces the desired outcome of an arrested cavity. If progress is not being made, I would assume this to mean that the necessary factors are not in place.

Studies have shown that nothing but unaltered saliva remineralized enamel cavities in one to four weeks.[41,42] I learned in dental school that three months is a good amount of time to attempt to remineralize a cavity, and I continue to follow such recommendations.[43] If successful remineralization is achieved, congratulations! If successful remineralization does not occur, three months is usually not enough time for more damage to occur. (Unless you have very rapidly progressing cavities, which is why you should get rapidly progressing cavities restored, and/or your dentist tells you serious damage could occur within three months.)

Assuming the cavity is an appropriate candidate for remineralization, the reason it might be taking a long time is not because the process of remineralization itself takes a long time, but because it is taking the person a long time to achieve the necessary conditions for remineralization.

Being educated about the details of cavity prevention and remineralization is your best course of action to minimize the risks, maximize the efficacy of your choices and bring you closer to having the mouth you desire.

# 3

# Reality TV Show
# &
# Cavities

"Undoubtedly, intact, nonrestored teeth are superior to restored teeth."

*— Sturdevant's Art & Science of Operative Dentistry* [1]

When I first met my husband, Andre, he was under the care of an excellent dentist in a lovely part of Toronto. (The only reason he no longer sees him is because we do not live in Toronto anymore.) Andre told me that his dentist told him he had little cavities in between all of his teeth. Yes, ALL of his teeth! The dentist told Andre that he and the hygienist would watch the cavities and hopefully they would harden. If they didn't, he would need fillings. After he left his appointment, Andre realized he'd forgotten to ask what he should do to help harden the cavities so they didn't progress. All he knew to do was to brush and floss, which he already did every day. Andre, like many others, asked me how to prevent and remineralize cavities. A common answer from the modern dental office is to use fluoride. There are many other ways to prevent and remineralize cavities, whether you want to use them in addition to or instead of fluoride. These additional ways will be discussed in the subsequent chapters of this book. First, in order to know how to prevent and remineralize cavities, it is necessary to know what causes a cavity.

## What Causes a Cavity?

In order for a cavity to occur, there needs to be three critical factors in place.[2]

1. Cavity-causing bacteria

2. Food for the cavity-causing bacteria

3. A susceptible tooth

**Susceptible Tooth + Cavity-Causing Bacteria
+ Food for Bacteria = Cavity**

**Healthy and Strong Tooth + Cavity-Causing Bacteria +
Food for Bacteria
= Greater Risk of Getting a Cavity, but No Cavity**

**Susceptible Tooth + No Cavity-Causing Bacteria
= Other Dental Problems
(Breakage, Sensitivity, Wear[3]) but No Cavity**

The first and second factors are obviously related; without food, the bacteria would die. For simplicity, from now on I refer to these two factors as the bacteria factor only.

A susceptible tooth is also necessary, for without a susceptible tooth, any amount of cavity-causing bacteria will be unable to cause a cavity. Cavity-causing bacteria is only cavity-*causing* in a susceptible tooth. A more accurate but cumbersome description would be cavity-causing-in-a-susceptible-tooth bacteria.

The twentieth and twenty-first centuries have seen much research regarding cavities and the cause of cavities. The conclusion from this research is that **both** internal and external factors are necessary for a cavity to develop. This means that both bacteria and a susceptible tooth need to be involved.[4] And doesn't this make logical sense? Many diseases and conditions require multiple factors to be present in order to be expressed, and often one of the factors involved is susceptibility and another factor is bacteria. For example, someone sneezes on an airplane. The same bacteria or virus is inhaled by many people – it is the person with the susceptible immune system (the internal factors) who comes down with the cold or flu.

Another example is a skin infection. Usually the bacterium, *Staphylococcus aureus* is said to cause the skin infection, but in reality the skin needed to be susceptible to the bacterium in order for infection to occur. Since 25% to 30% of the population has *Staphylococcus aureus* on their skin without even knowing it, it is especially clear that only those individuals with susceptible skin and bodies will experience the problems of a 'staph infection.'

**Bacteria/Virus + Susceptible Individual = Cold/Flu**

**S. aureus + Susceptible Skin = Skin Infection**

**Bacteria + Susceptible Tooth = Cavity**

Let's pretend we have created a new reality TV show. The contestants have to build a house or some sort of structure and the person whose structure lasts the longest wins a lot of money. The contestants can choose to build their house in any part of the world with any materials they choose. The buildings will then be put to the test with the most harsh simulated environmental conditions a house might be exposed to in that particular part of the world.

If you were a contestant, what will you do to try to win? Well of course you will build a house using the strongest possible materials and put it in a part of the world exposed to the least harsh environment. You know that building a house out of Popsicle sticks in a tornado zone is going to make you a star on the TV show, but not from winning any money!

Let's say on our new reality TV show the contestants have a limited amount time to build their structure. Some chose to spend all their time focusing on strong materials. They didn't travel anywhere else in the world, they just made super strong houses out of incredibly strong materials; steel beams, concrete walls and reinforced trusses. These contestants thought for sure they were going to win – how could they not with such strong houses? But they didn't take into consideration the environment at all, and since the filming takes place near the ocean, the TV producers simulated a flood and the host showed the houses floating atop water. No win for the strong houses.

The next few contestants decided to build their structures in parts of the world that are not exposed to harsh climates and risk factors. They spent so much time getting to their locations – flying out, waiting in airports for transfers, even traveling on camel or moped to get to their ideal spot, by the time they arrived there was little time to build a house. Sourcing strong materials in these exotic locations was impossible, so they ended up with poorly made houses. Even though the weak houses were in serene environmental climates, the creative TV producers found a way to destroy the houses. (Hey, this is sounding like a good TV show the more I write!) They sent in a group of teenagers to play basketball in the front of the house, and in no time at all, the force of the basketball banging against the walls knocked these contestants out of the competition.

The winner was someone who had both a strong house and calm environmental conditions. The person traveled a little away but not very far and had plenty of time for building a house out of strong materials.

The factors necessary for having long-lasting, healthy teeth are actually quite similar to building a long-lasting house. There are environmental factors as well as structural factors.

## Environmental Factors:

Environmental factors for teeth are the conditions occurring within the mouth.

## A Harsh or Helpful Environment

- pH
- Bacteria
- Saliva

## Structural or Internal Factors:

Structural factors for teeth are the conditions within the body affecting the internal state and structural integrity of teeth.

## A Strong or Susceptible Tooth

- Matrix Metalloproteinases
- Hormones
- Dentin Fluid Flow
- Autonomic Nervous System
- Food

A tooth that is very strong with a low susceptibility but has a harsh mouth environment is like the strong houses built in a flood zone. A weak and susceptible tooth in a mouth consisting of a serene or helpful environment is like the poorly made houses in perfect environmental conditions. People who have susceptible teeth in a harsh mouth environment are in a situation like the contestant who made a house out of Popsicle sticks in a hurricane zone.

While the houses and the teeth that have good structural factors but bad environmental factors fare much better than the Popsicle stick house in a hurricane, these houses and teeth are not without problems, or increased risk of problems. Likewise, the houses and teeth that have good environmental conditions but weak structure do better than the Popsicle stick house in a hurricane, but these houses and teeth are also not without problems and increased risk of problems.

Clearly, it is ideal to address all the factors involved with cavities. Sure it is possible to be cavity-free by only addressing the environmental factors or by only addressing the susceptibility or internal factors, but I assure you that both your overall and oral health will be superior if you address both internal and environmental factors, particularly if you use natural approaches.

Even though I separate the environmental and susceptibility/internal factors, they are indeed intricately related with overlap. Just like with building a house, the two factors greatly affect each other. For example, even though I say the materials used to construct a house are categorized as a structural factor, the choice of materials to select from is dictated by the part of the world where the house is being made, thus the structural factors are not at all separate from the environmental factors. This is the same with cavities. I separate the factors into different categories because I think it makes them easier to explain and conceptualize, but in reality they are all related. For example, the same food that will affect the environmental factors of pH and saliva, will also affect the susceptibility or internal factors of dentinal fluid flow, MMPs and hormones.

I often hear people discuss the susceptibility factor as if nothing can be done to change it. "I just have soft teeth," "cavities run in my family," "I get bad/good teeth from my mom," are all examples of the idea that a susceptible tooth is determined by genetics and is unchangeable. While genetics does play a role, and the structure of one's teeth developed in utero and in childhood has an impact on tooth susceptibility later in life, there is much that can be done in the present moment to improve resistance and decrease susceptibility to cavities.

Unlike the fictitious reality TV show where only one person can be a winner, thankfully in reality everyone can be a winner with healthy, cavity-free teeth!

By the way, all of Andre's tiny cavities hardened up!

# 4

---

# A Harsh or Helpful Environment: pH

"No longer is restoration of a carious lesion considered a cure."

— *Sturdevant's Art & Science of Operative Dentistry*[1]

Imagine your child coming up to you and saying, "Mommy or Daddy, my mouth is growing cavities right now. I need my special drink to stop them." You give them their requested drink and then they say, "Oh good. Cavities stopped. Thank you, Mommy or Daddy."

Does that sound like a dream? Having a young child know when cavities are at risk of occurring in their mouth and how to alleviate that risk – that dream can be a reality and I have seen it happen! It is a reality made possible by teaching your child how to measure their mouth pH. Measuring mouth pH is so incredibly easy and provides such powerful information. Children find it fun! Children get to spit and then watch a piece of paper turn colour – and parents get to know whether their mouth environment is in a harsh or helpful state. It's like a dream come true for everyone!

## pH 101

pH is a measurement of acid. Just like milliliters and ounces measure liquids and kilometers and miles measure distance, pH measures acid. pH, which stands for power or potentiation of hydrogen, measures the concentration of hydrogen ions in a solution. Hydrogen ions (H+) are extremely acidic. The higher the concentration, the more acidic the solution; the lower the concentration, the more basic or alkaline the solution. Basic and alkaline mean the same thing.

The pH measurement scale generally goes from 1 to 14. In dentistry, pH is measured to one decimal point, and the scale usually only ranges from pH 5 to 8. While that may seem like a very small range compared to other measurements, each number represents a huge change in acidity. For example, the difference between pH 6 and pH 7 is that pH 6 has ten times the concentration of hydrogen ions and is ten times as acidic as pH 7. The greater the number of hydrogen ions, the lower the pH number.

**High hydrogen, high acidity = low pH number**

**pH 7 = neutral (not acidic and not alkaline)**

**pH less than 7 = acidic**

**pH greater than 7 = alkaline/basic**

# Acid Dissolves Enamel

pH is an important concept for remineralization of teeth because in the presence of acid, minerals dissolve out of the tooth.

Remember that enamel and dentin are made up of the molecule, hydroxyapatite. Hydroxyapatite is composed of calcium, phosphate and hydroxyl. (The chemical composition of hydroxyapatite is: $Ca_{10}(PO_4)_6(OH)_2$.)

Ca = Calcium

$PO_4$ = phosphate

OH = hydroxyl

Phosphate and hydroxyl can both be altered in the presence of hydrogen (H+) ions. Phosphate becomes hydroxy phosphate but is still usually called phosphate. Hydroxyl (OH) combines with hydrogen (H+) to become HOH, otherwise known as $H_2O$ or water. The desire or affinity of hydrogen to combine with OH to become $H_2O$ is very strong, and as such, in the presence of hydrogen (acidity), the OH would much rather form water than stay in the hydroxyapatite molecule. This means that the hydroxyapatite molecule is broken apart, or is dissolved, in the presence of hydrogen (acidity). No longer does the enamel contain that molecule of hydroxyapatite, and the saliva now contains a water molecule, a calcium mineral and a phosphate.

In the presence of acidic saliva – a high number of hydrogen (H+) ions which means a pH lower than 7 – the following occurs:

**In the saliva: - Calcium**

**- Phosphate**

**- Water**

**(Hydroxyapatite no longer in enamel)**

In the presence of neutral or alkaline saliva – a low number of hydrogen (H+) ions which means a pH of 7 or higher – the following occurs:

**In the enamel:**

**Hydroxyapatite**

# The Critical pH

pH 5.5 is called the critical pH, where the concentration of hydrogen ions is so great that enough hydroxyapatite is dissolved to form a cavity. pH 5.5 is not good. If you or your child see a pH score of 5.5, you should treat it like a mini emergency situation and take action to raise mouth pH immediately.

However, pH 5.5 is not the only pH capable of causing a cavity. Cavities can occur at a higher pH as well, depending on the number of calcium and phosphate ions present in the saliva. If calcium and phosphate levels are low in the saliva, the hydroxyapatite has a greater desire or affinity to break apart to provide the deficient calcium and phosphate to the saliva in an effort to balance out the differing concentrations. This means that fewer hydrogen ions are required in order to break apart or dissolve the hydroxyapatite, and it can occur at a pH higher than 5.5.[2] In a mineral-deficient mouth, less acidity is capable of causing a cavity.

Therefore, to ensure teeth are in a state of remineralization and not demineralization, it is best to maintain saliva at a neutral pH or as close to neutral as possible (pH 7). Some people think that since pH 7 is good, higher must be even better, but this is not the case. It is not necessary or even healthy to strive to have a much higher pH than neutral.

Recap:

pH scale usually goes from 1 to 14 and each number represents a huge change in acidity. Right in the middle of the scale is 7, which represents a neutral solution, which means it is neither acidic nor alkaline. Alkaline or basic is the opposite of acidic. Any number that is higher than 7 is alkaline. Any number below 7 is acidic.

So let's have a little test:

· If your saliva is pH 7, what is happening to your teeth? The minerals are in hydroxyapatite and your teeth are strong – excellent!

· If your saliva is pH 5.5, what is happening to your teeth? The minerals would rather form water in the saliva than stay in hydroxyapatite, so the minerals dissolve out of your teeth. Demineralization is occurring and the cavity process is in place – not a good situation.

· If your saliva is pH 6.5 and you are deficient in minerals, what is happening to your teeth? The minerals would rather be in the saliva to balance the concentration difference than stay in hydroxyapatite, so the minerals dissolve out of the teeth. Demineralization is occurring and the cavity process is in place – not a good situation.

## How to Know if Your Mouth is Acidic

You can easily determine if your mouth is in an acidic state. You can purchase pH paper inexpensively online or at some health food and grocery stores. It is best to purchase pH paper that indicates pH to one decimal point. For example, it is ideal to be able to see whether your saliva is pH 6.6, 6.7, 6.8, 6.9, etc. Some pH strips will indicate every other decimal point, such as 6.6, 6.8, 7.0, etc., and this is good as well. If the scale does not include decimal points and goes from 5 to 6 to 7, this is fine to purchase as a last resort, but you will not be able to determine as much detailed and useful information – there is quite a difference between 6.1 and 6.9.

The pH paper will come with a color-coded chart that should only be used with the pH strips it came with, as every company and even different papers within a company will have different color-coded charts associated with pH values.

Children usually have fun testing their mouth pH, and often are able to do so by themselves with some instruction. Even infants usually tolerate testing very well.

## How to Test

Spit into a cup or pool some saliva in your mouth, then put a strip in the pooled saliva. Make sure the strip is covered entirely with saliva. A partially covered strip will give an inaccurate result. Quickly remove the strip from your mouth or cup and immediately compare the strip to the color chart. Do not let the strip sit for any length of time before or during comparing to the color chart because the color will change with time and can give you a falsely alkaline number. Discard the strip as they cannot be reused. Also note that the strips must be discarded if they get any water on them, so be sure to keep the package away from water or other liquids.

To test an infant or young child's pH, put the paper into their mouth, touching either their cheek or tongue. You can also put the pH paper into their drool.

## When to Test

Salivary pH is completely unique to the individual, and can change multiple times per day. Children can have different pH levels than parents; foods and drinks can affect people differently or even the same person differently during different stages of their life, or even day.

I highly recommend testing yours or your child's mouth pH very often for at least two days, after which it is not necessary to continue with such rigorous testing. Once you figure out any potential problem times, you can simply focus on testing pH during those times.

## Schedule

Record pH for the following times:

Upon waking: _____

After breakfast: _____

After coffee or mid-morning snack: _____

Immediately before lunch (or a time when no food or drink has been had for an hour or more): _____

After lunch: _____

After afternoon snack: _____

Immediately prior to dinner (or a time when no food or drink has been had for an hour or more): _____

After dinner: _____

Before brushing teeth: _____

After brushing teeth and right before going to sleep: _____

## Interpreting Your Results

Here are some example scenarios you may discover and how to deal with them: (Please note these are only very general guidelines and may not apply to you specifically.)

# If you find acidic saliva...

## After Certain Foods

If you consistently have neutral saliva but noticed that your mouth is acidic after eating or drinking certain foods, this is actually a fairly simple issue to improve, and will have substantial benefits. One of the reasons I love recommending testing mouth pH is because it allows people to learn so much about their bodies. While there are lists of foods that are generally considered acidic and foods that are generally considered alkaline, these foods can affect individuals differently. People always ask me if their favorite drinks or foods are acidic. "Is coffee acidic?" "Is lemon water acidic?" "Is an apple acidic?" To know for sure, all you have to do is check! If you notice your mouth is acidic after a certain food or drink, then either stop consuming that food or drink, or follow it with something that is neutral or alkaline and then re-test your mouth to make sure it has neutralized. For example, if you notice that coffee leaves your mouth acidic, then you definitely don't want to be sipping on coffee all day long. Instead, either stop the all-day coffee or follow it with a food or drink that will neutralize it.

Do Not Brush Your Teeth While Acidic!

The first thing many people want to do when they see an acidic result on the pH strip is to brush their teeth. While it is true that brushing your teeth with toothpaste will probably raise the pH of your mouth (toothpastes are usually neutral or alkaline), it is not the best way to do so. Teeth are in a vulnerable state in an acidic mouth and scrubbing away at the enamel in this vulnerable state can result in more loss of enamel. Loss of enamel from excessive wear and abrasion are common problems experienced by people today, and brushing teeth while the mouth is acidic can be a contributing factor.

## Neutral Foods and Drinks

The way to neutralize something acidic is to combine it with something neutral or alkaline. I like to think of acid as scalding-hot water, something alkaline as ice water and something neutral as room-temperature water. You want to take a drink of water but your water is scalding hot (acidic). How can you cool it down? You can combine it with some ice water (alkaline). You probably don't need too much ice water to cool it down. Or you can cool it down by combining the scalding-hot water with room-temperature water. If you only add a small amount of room-temperature water, you won't cool it down very much. You need a lot of room-temperature water. This is the same with having acid in your mouth. You can get rid of the acidity by either adding something alkaline or neutral. You won't need too much of the alkaline substance, but you will need a lot of the neutral substance. As acidity increases, it is like the water becomes even hotter, and more cooling substances are needed. The more acidic the mouth, the more alkaline and even more neutral substances are needed to offset it.

Speaking of water, it is often a neutral substance and can be enough for some people to neutralize their mouth with. However, other people will require something more alkaline than water to neutralize their mouth, just like hot-water requires a more alkaline substance than room-temperature water to neutralize it. Also, sometimes water does not have a neutral pH. If you aren't sure whether water will neutralize your mouth, all you have to do is check your pH.

## If you find acidic saliva...

## Upon Waking

If you consistently have neutral saliva but notice that your mouth is acidic when you wake up, this may seem like an easy problem to correct, but may in fact be quite a challenge – but, of course, worth the effort. It's possible that your mouth is in an acidic state all night long. Sleeping creates a harsh environment for teeth, because of the greatly reduced amount of saliva produced. Low levels of saliva combined with an acidic mouth make for an incredibly harsh environment.

A very common cause of acidity during the night is mouth breathing. At rest, our lips should be closed, with teeth slightly open. This allows for adequate levels of saliva to be maintained in the mouth, and for the self-cleansing actions of saliva to take place. If someone habitually breathes through their mouth and their lips remain apart at rest, they are said to be mouth breathing or to be a mouth breather. It is ideal to breathe through the nose, not the mouth. Obviously, if someone is sick with a congested nose and it temporarily results in mouth breathing, this would not put the person at the same level of risk as chronic mouth breathing does. I do, however, find mouth breathing to be quite common for many people, at least during some parts of the year, and often for much of their life.

There are many causes of mouth breathing, a common one being allergies. People sometimes take allergies lightly and shrug them off as humorous. "I know I'm allergic to cats but I have four," type of thinking. I strongly urge people to get their allergies under control. In addition, mouth breathing in children will often result in jaw constrictions, necessitating the need for orthodontics.[3] If mouth breathing continues or begins in adulthood, people who have had orthodontics experience a higher degree of relapse, and their teeth move back out of alignment. Mouth breathing is associated with decreased IQ, hyperactivity in children, fatigue in adults, hypertension and overall decreased oxygen to the brain.[4,5,6,7,8,9,10,11]

If you or your child has allergies, go for allergy testing or somehow figure out what the allergen is. It is very common for people to be allergic to or have reactions to gluten and dairy. If hay fever, ragweed, dust, pollen or other ubiquitous things are causing problems, then I suggest getting to the root of the problem, which is an overactive immune system. See a healthcare professional to help improve the function of your immune system, perhaps by diet changes, detoxification and other lifestyle modifications.

In addition to decreasing mouth breathing and/or if you don't mouth breath, here are some other ideas to keep your mouth hydrated and neutral all night long.

a) Increase fluid intake (without caffeine) before bedtime or even during the day.

b) Make sure you go to bed with your mouth in an alkaline state. Give it the best chance possible to be neutral all night by starting off alkaline.

## If you find acidic saliva...

## During the Day

If you consistently have neutral saliva but noticed that your mouth is acidic during the day or part of the day, this is actually a fairly simple issue to improve, and will have substantial benefits. If you are able to achieve neutral saliva during some of the more challenging times of the day, like upon waking, you will most likely be able to achieve neutral saliva during the day as well.

Two common causes of acidic saliva during the day are dehydration and stress.

# Dehydration

A dry mouth automatically drops the pH of the mouth and makes it more acidic.

## Dry Mouth = More Acidic

Here's how:

Saliva naturally contains alkaline, baking-soda-like molecules called bicarbonate, to neutralize acidity.

Yes, our body produces baking-soda-like molecules to neutralize our mouth! Bicarbonate has a pH of about 9.

Bicarbonate $= HCO_3-$

(Baking soda = Sodium with Bicarbonate $= NaHCO_3$)

Let's say that Joe, our fictitious busy man has found that he consistently has acidic saliva every day in the afternoon. For the purpose of this example, let's pretend that Joe's saliva contains 4 bicarbonate molecules per 1 mL of saliva.

4 molecules:1 mL

Sometimes during the day, like after eating or drinking, Joe has 1 mL of saliva in his mouth. How many neutralizing bicarbonate molecules does he have? Four. And that is enough to result in neutralization and his pH strips show a neutral result.

In the afternoons, however, Joe is so busy working that he has no time to take a break and drink anything. When he is dehydrated, he only has 0.25 mL of saliva in his mouth. So now how many neutralizing bicarbonate molecules does he have?

4:1mL

x:0.25mL

x=1

One bicarbonate is not enough to neutralize his mouth, leaving his mouth acidic. The pH strip shows a number less than 7.

Joe does have protective saliva, just not enough of it during certain parts of the day.


## Stress

Another common reason people experience a drop in pH and increase in acidity during the day is stress. Stress results in less saliva production.[12] The body focuses on other physiological processes that will aid it in dealing with the stress, and saliva is not something that will help one deal with an emergency situation. A decrease in saliva production will automatically drop the pH of the saliva, as seen in the above example.

If you can't eliminate or decrease your stress then at least make sure you are well hydrated and drinking enough fluids to keep your mouth neutral all day long. The last thing you need is the extra stress of dental problems!

## If you find acidic saliva...

## All the Time

If you consistently have acidic saliva, you have just made a huge discovery for yourself, and now have the amazing opportunity to dramatically improve your life. By changing your saliva from consistently acidic to consistently neutral you will not only experience a great improvement in your oral health, but you will also reap great systemic benefits.[13]

If you consistently have acidic saliva, you may have any of the above mentioned issues, just happening all day long. For example, you may be mouth breathing all day long, eating acidic foods all day long, experiencing dehydration all day long or have chronic stress. Having consistently acidic saliva sometimes happens in certain disease states, such as hypothyroidism,[14] diabetes, Sjögren's Syndrome, chronic infections and salivary gland pathology.[15] If you have or think you might have a systemic concern, it is best to seek the advice of a healthcare professional.

Here are some ways to raise the pH of your saliva. It is best to find ways that are enjoyable to you so you can keep the changes long term.

## a) Incorporate More Greens Into Your Diet

What makes green plants green is a molecule called chlorophyll. Chlorophyll has a pH of about 11. Eating more green vegetables will help increase the pH of your mouth,[16] and will also be great for the rest of your body.

Here are some examples of how to incorporate more greens into your diet:

-Juicing

-Green Smoothies

-Sea Veggies

-Salads

Also, you can purchase chlorophyll on its own. Chlorophyll comes as a liquid and you can put drops of it into water. It does turn the water green, but most people, including children, usually don't mind the taste of a few drops of chlorophyll in their water. You can put anywhere from a few drops to a teaspoon of chlorophyll in water, put less for children. However, I wouldn't rely on chlorophyll drops as your main source of chlorophyll. Consuming the majority of it as a whole food in vegetables is best. Chlorophyll drops can also be added to water and used like a mouthwash.

## b) Homemade Mouthwash[17]

1 teaspoon salt
1 teaspoon baking soda
1 cup water

You can also add baking soda to toothpaste or onto a toothbrush. Note that brushing with baking soda is abrasive on the teeth and should not be done if wear or erosion are concerns. Instead of brushing, swishing and spitting is an alternative.

## c) Milk of Magnesia[18,19]

Swish and spit out, like a mouthwash.

## d) Minerals[20]

Add a few drops of a liquid mineral supplement to drinking water.

# Buffering Capacity

Buffering capacity is the ability of the saliva to neutralize acid. Buffering capacity, while related to pH, is different in that pH is the level of acid found in someone's mouth at any given time, while buffering capacity is an intrinsic factor that plays a major role in determining the resultant pH of someone's mouth.

For example, some people can drink an acidic substance, like pop, and test their mouth pH a moment later to find their mouth neutral. Other people will take more time to neutralize their mouth acidity – like a few minutes, and others still will take hours or never neutralize their mouth.

People with a highly effective buffering capacity/capability will have a lowered risk of cavities. Not zero risk, of course, due to the other factors involved with cavity formation, but certainly their teeth will be exposed to much less acid than someone with a poor buffering capacity, meaning a cavity will be less likely to form.

Remember, the buffering ability of saliva is primarily completed by action of bicarbonate ions. The greater the concentration of bicarbonate ions, the greater the ability of the saliva to neutralize acidic conditions in the mouth.[21]

## How to Know Your Buffering Capacity

Tests are available at your dentist's office to measure buffering capacity. You can also get an idea of your buffering capacity by doing the following test at home.

Directions:

Select an acidic liquid of your choice: apple juice, lemon juice or vinegar. You may choose another liquid as long as the pH is below 5.5.

Swish with a teaspoon of your acidic drink for 20 seconds. After spitting the drink out, check your mouth pH.

If the pH strip is neutral you may stop.

If you do not have neutral saliva, pretend to chew something while running your tongue over your teeth. Do this for one minute and check your saliva again. If the pH strip is neutral you may stop.

If you still have acidic pH, continue making chewing motions and running your tongue over your teeth. Check your pH every minute until you have neutral pH.

After five minutes, check one last time. If you still have acidic saliva, stop the process and drink some water, water with chlorophyll drops or a drink of your choice that you have found to make your mouth neutral.

Compare the time it took for your saliva to neutralize acid to the following chart to get an idea of what your buffering capacity is:

**Immediately (within the first 20 seconds): Very High**

**1 minute later: High**

**2 minutes later: Moderate**

**3 minutes later: Low**

**4 minutes later: Low**

**5 minutes later or not at all: Very Low**

## Manually Neutralize Your Mouth

The benefit of getting your buffering capacity tested at your dentist's office and/or doing the above test, is to know whether buffering capacity is your Achilles' heel. If you find that you have poor buffering capacity, you know this is an area that you cannot slack on. While your friend might be able to drink lemon water or honey-sweetened tea with no adverse consequences, if you have low buffering capacity, you will know that instead of relying on your saliva to neutralize an acidic drink or food, you need to manually neutralize it yourself. There is no need to stop drinking acidic foods and drinks since many healthy substances can produce acid in one's mouth; you simply need to take an extra step to neutralize the acid. I call this, manually neutralizing your mouth. Use pH paper to learn which foods and drinks are best to neutralize your mouth with, and use these foods and drinks as your go-to after meals and snacks.

## How to Naturally Improve Buffering Capacity

Our body naturally produces bicarbonate, not only for our mouth, but for the rest of the body. Bicarbonate is essential to regulate the pH of our interstitial fluids and tissues, urine, and most important of all, our blood. Blood must be at a critical pH (arterial blood = 7.41) or else serious systemic concerns will occur.[22] Blood takes precedence over the saliva, and if bicarbonate is needed to keep the blood pH within normal range, and there is not enough left over for the saliva, so be it. The teeth suffer. This is actually a good thing – the body has its priorities straight! But how about having both the blood *and* the saliva in optimal conditions? That would be ideal, right? It is possible.

In addition to genetics, there are numerous factors that could result in a reduced level of bicarbonate ions in our saliva. An increase in acid in the body (using up sources of bicarbonate to keep the blood in the critical range of pH) or a loss of bicarbonate would have the overall effect of diminished buffering capacity in the mouth.

**More Acid in Body**

**= More Bicarbonate Used to Neutralize**

**= Less Bicarbonate for the Mouth**

**= Acidic Mouth**

**&**

**Loss of Bicarbonate From Body**

**= Less Bicarbonate for the Mouth**

**= Acidic Mouth**


Action Steps

**1. Increase bicarbonate intake**

- Naturally occurring bicarbonate is found in natural spring water.

- Sodium bicarbonate is baking soda. For a transient increase in the concentration of bicarbonate in one's saliva, use baking soda as a mouthrinse or toothpaste.[23]

## 2. Decrease Body's Need for Bicarbonate

- Avoid toxins. Exposure to toxins such as ethylene glycol (antifreeze), paraldehyde (preservative), and ammonium chloride use up bicarbonate so less is available in the saliva.[24]

Ammonium chloride sources:

- Food additive (E510)

- Gives baked goods crisp texture

- Feed supplement for cattle

- Fertilizer, especially for rice and wheat grown in Asia

- Thickener in shampoo

- Cough medicine

- Cleaning products

## 3. Improve digestion and gut health[25]

## 4. Reduce lactic acid build up (such as by staying fit)[26]

## 5. Ensure well regulated disease states (such as diabetes and kidney disease)[27]

Buffering capacity does not change frequently like pH can. Improving your buffering capacity will require great time and effort, after which it still might not even change. I recommend focusing daily on improving your pH, which will be far easier to improve. Improving your buffering capacity can be a long-term goal for the future. Certainly taking positive steps to improve your buffering capacity daily is a great idea, but expecting it to change in a matter of days or months is not realistic.

So often people ask me in passing or when there is just a moment of time, how to naturally prevent and remineralize cavities. Clearly I do not think there is an answer to that question that can be said in just a moment's time, since I have written an entire book on the subject! However, if I absolutely must answer in a brief passing moment, I tell people to purchase some pH paper and check their saliva. Checking salivary pH is well received by many people, and is such a powerful tool that it is my quick go-to answer. There is simply no other prevention and remineralization strategy for kids (and some adults!) that is as fun as being told to spit on a color-changing paper.

# 5

# A Harsh or Helpful Environment: Bacteria

"The specific plaque hypothesis provides a new scientific basis for the treatment of caries that has radically altered caries treatment."

*— Sturdevant's Art & Science of Operative Dentistry[1]*

Although there are many factors that contribute to the cause of a cavity, bacteria is a huge and major factor. Remember the modern definition of a cavity is that it is an infectious disease caused by bacteria that produce acid which demineralizes the teeth. Of course, there are the internal susceptibility factors, but a cavity does not occur there is the presence of cavity-causing bacteria.[2,3] For example, demineralization or the removal of minerals without the presence of cavity-causing bacteria will result in wear, erosion, abrasion or some other dental problems, but not an active cavity.[4]

There are over 300 species of microorganisms found in the mouth, most of which are incapable of creating a cavity.[5] The genus, *Streptococcus*, refers to the shape of certain bacteria (circular-shaped) which many different species fall under. Of those many species, there is only one group of bacteria that is capable of starting a cavity. This group of bacteria is called, *Streptococcus mutans*, and *Streptococcus mutans* consists of eight serotypes, or 'sub-groups,' such as *Streptococcus rattus, Streptococcus ferus* and *Streptococcus sangria. Strepococcus mutans* is the most commonly discussed cavity-causing bacteria, and is sometimes abbreviated to *S. mutans* or Strep mutans. The collective group of cavity-initiating bacteria are sometimes called Mutans Streptococci or MS bacteria, which refers to all the different species that are cavity-causing.[6]

*Streptococcus mutans* = **Strep mutans,** *S. mutans*

**= Most Commonly Known Cavity-Causing Bacteria**

**Mutans Streptococci = MS bacteria = Group of Cavity-Causing Bacteria, including** *Streptococcus mutans*

Throughout this book, when I refer to cavity-causing bacteria, I am referring to Mutans Streptococci (MS), which includes *Streptococcus mutans.*

Most people have at least some MS bacteria in their mouth, which is not surprising because over 90% of the population have cavities. Numerous studies have shown that the more MS bacteria in one's mouth, the more cavities are present, and the greater the risk of getting a cavity in the future.[7,8] It is possible to have a high level of MS bacteria and not have active cavities, but one is considered to be at high risk and more susceptible to cavities.

# How to Reduce Cavity-Causing Bacteria

Clearly, it is advantageous to reduce the levels of cavity-causing or MS bacteria in one's mouth. One of the ways to reduce bad bacteria levels is reduce *all* bacteria levels. It is not possible to completely sterilize the mouth, however, lowering levels of all bacteria will in effect lower levels of MS or cavity-causing bacteria. Brushing, flossing and antimicrobial rinses like chlorhexidine function to lower the overall level of bacteria in the mouth.

The following have also been shown to reduce levels of oral bacteria:

1. **Lauric acid** has been shown to reduce oral bacteria including *Streptococcus mutans*.[9] Lauric acid is plentiful in coconut oil and milk.

2. **Iodine**.[10] Iodine has antimicrobial properties and has been shown to reduce levels of *Streptococcus mutans* when applied topically as a mouthrinse.[11,12,13] Povidone-iodine applied to children's teeth three times over a six-month period resulted in a reduction of new cavity development compared to controls.[14]

3. **Cheese** has been shown to reduce incidence of cavities, and one of several reasons is thought to be because of the ability to reduce adhesion of bacteria.[15]

4. **Bioflavonoids** are a class of antioxidants which are plentiful in grapes and grape products. Grape seed extract and raisons have been tested and found to be effective against oral bacteria, including *Streptococcus mutans*.[16] Bioflavonoids are effective at eliminating bacteria because bioflavonoids inhibit glucosyltransferases. Glucosyltransferases are produced by bacteria, including MS bacteria, and are used during the pro-

cess of creating glucans, which help the bacteria adhere to teeth and form plaque. [17, 18]

Sources of flavonoids:[19]

- Fruits, especially citrus, apples, red grapes, berries

- Vegetables, especially onions

- Tea leaves

- Plant barks, leaves, rinds, seeds and flowers

5. **Clove** compounds have been found to inhibit the growth of oral pathogens.[20] Clove is a component of the dental material, ZOE (Zinc Oxide Eugenol), which is often used for temporary fillings when the pulp is irritated. The filling is done as an attempt to heal the pulp and avoid needing a root canal.[21] You can add clove powder or clove oil onto your toothbrush and use it to brush your teeth.

6. *Ceanothus americanus* is a shrub native to North America. The plant has traditionally been used as a tea to treat upper respiratory infections by native populations. Today it is known as: New Jersey tea, red root tea, mountain sweet tea and wild snowball tea.[22] Laboratory studies have shown that *Ceanothus americanus* has antimicrobial abilities against oral pathogens, including S*treptococcus mutans*.[23]

7. **Chewing sticks** of the shrub, *Diospyros lycioides*, or muthala, known as the Namibia chewing stick have been shown to

exhibit significant growth inhibition of oral bacteria, including MS bacteria.[24,25]

**8. Goldenseal** (*Hydrastis canadensis*) is a popular herbal supplement often used as a cold/flu remedy. Components of goldenseal have been shown in laboratory studies to be an effective antimicrobial agent against oral bacteria, including *Streptococcus mutans*.[26,27]

**9. Liquorice root** *(Glycyrrhiza uralensis)* has been shown to reduce levels of *Streptococcus mutans*.[28]

**10. Xylitol** is a sugar substitute that has been shown to decrease levels of oral bacteria, including *Streptococcus mutans*. It is thought that xylitol's ability to decrease bacteria levels is due to its molecular structure. Xylitol is composed of 5 hydroxyl groups (OH groups) as opposed to the usual 6 hydroxyl groups that sugar and other sugar substitutes are composed of. Thus, xylitol is very similar to other sugars, but that one missing hydroxyl means bacteria can't use it as a fuel source.[29] When bacteria attempt to use xylitol as a fuel source, they end up dying because the altered composition of xylitol renders it ineffective. It is as if the xylitol tricks the bacteria into consuming it, like the witch tricked Snow White into eating a poisonous apple. If you wish to use xylitol as part of your prevention and remineralization strategy, you can make your own xylitol mouthwash with 1 cup of water and 1 to 2 tablespoons of xylitol. Swish with the mouthwash at least twice a day.

**Natural Approaches & Frequency**

Although it may seem appealing to use natural approaches for bacteria reduction, natural approaches must be used frequently and in high amounts in order to provide any effective actions. Using natural approaches once in a blue moon or whenever you remember will obviously not do any harm, but will also not really provide any real benefit. I suggest adding natural antibacterial products into your daily routine alongside brushing and flossing to ensure the most effective actions.

# Targeting the Cavity-Causing/ MS Bacteria

Dental plaque is that soft white goo that feels like your teeth are fuzzy. When plaque is removed, your teeth feel clean and shiny. It is "a gelatinous mass of bacteria adhering to the tooth surface."[30]

The Specific Plaque Hypothesis is significantly different than the Non-Specific Plaque Hypothesis, which assumes that all plaque is pathogenic and necessary for removal.

The Specific Plaque Hypothesis is based on the idea that **not all bacteria and not all plaque is bad** and necessary to remove. The goal within the Specific Plaque Hypothesis is to remove pathogenic organisms only, and to replace them with non-pathogenic organisms and plaque.[31] The Specific Plaque Hypothesis recognizes that not only is it impossible to remove all bacteria and sterilize the mouth, but it is actually not ideal, since non-pathogenic bacteria can actually be protective to teeth.[32] For example, studies have shown that teeth colonized by *Streptococcus mutans* are more likely to develop cavities, and teeth colonized by *Streptococcus sanguis*, which are incapable of causing a cavity, are more likely to be healthy and cavity-free.[33]

Removing MS bacteria and replacing them with non-MS bacteria is the objective for creating a helpful (as opposed to harmful) mouth environment.[34] Removing cavity-causing bacteria and replacing them with non-pathogenic organisms means the mouth needs to be *recolonized*.

## First Colonization

As soon as the deciduous or baby teeth erupt into a child's mouth, the teeth are immediately colonized by bacteria. Likewise, when the permanent or adult teeth first erupt, they are also immediately colonized by bacteria. Colonization means "to inhabit, cultivate, tend to and guard."[35] Colonization is like being covered by bacteria, but even more long term. Colonies of bacteria are highly organized, and the bacteria which first colonize a tooth set up to live there long term, and are said to create a sort of bacteria plug that protects them from being taken over by another type of bacteria.[36] Generation after generation of bacteria are reproduced, and so even though some bacteria die or are eliminated, the same type of bacteria will be found on the tooth where the initial colonization took place.[37,38] The types of bacteria that are prevalent in the mouth at the time of tooth eruption determines the types of bacteria doing the early colonization of teeth. The bacteria that colonize the mouth and teeth have developed resistance to the antimicrobial components in saliva.[39]

It is highly advantageous to have your teeth colonized by non-MS or non-cavity-causing bacteria. Since bacteria greatly resist an introduction of new bacteria – or a changeover of colonizers of the teeth – one will be significantly protected from cavities by starting out with non-MS bacteria. Not only will these bacteria be incapable of creating a cavity, but they will actually resist the invasion of MS or cavity-causing bacteria. The non-MS bacteria will be working hard to protect you from cavities, and you don't even realize it or have to do anything.

## Children and Infants

Some people have heard that cavities are an infectious disease and that parents can pass it to their children. This is referring to the fact that MS or cavity-causing bacteria need to get into one's mouth somehow, and if a parent kisses their child this would be a way to pass along the MS or bad bacteria. (There are still the tooth susceptibility factors to address, which are covered in subsequent chapters.)

Instead of avoiding kissing your child – who wants to do that! – reduce your levels of bad bacteria and you can kiss your child all you want, hopefully passing along some good and protective bacteria!

**Did You Know?**
Which bacteria will initially colonize a baby is determined before the baby is even born. While it has historically been thought that babies are born with sterile guts, new studies have shown that babies are born with bacteria already existing in their gut, and that the bacteria closely resembles the bacteria in the mother's mouth![40] Clearly our gut and our mouths are intricately linked from very early on.

# How to Recolonize the Mouth

Bacteria in the mouth get rid of each other by out-producing and creating greater numbers than the others, and occupying all the living space. With nothing to eat and nowhere to live, the old bacteria die off and the new bacteria take over and re-colonize the teeth.[41] Many types of bacteria are capable of killing MS bacteria, and therefore resist the creation of a cavity.[42,43] Introducing very high numbers of these types of bacteria will result in the recolonization of teeth, and the transformation of the mouth environment from one that is harsh (containing cavity-causing bacteria) to one that is helpful (containing cavity-resisting bacteria). Recolonizing your mouth with cavity-resisting bacteria is a highly effective form of protection from cavities.

# Action Steps:

## 1. Consume Probiotic Foods

Fermented foods utilize bacteria or other microorganisms to produce the resultant characteristic food product. Examples of such foods include yogurt, cheese, sour cream, pickles and sauerkraut. Several strains of bacteria found in fermented foods have been shown to be able to recolonize the mouth and resist the colonization of MS or cavity-causing bacteria (as well as bacteria associated with gum disease[44,45] and bad breath[46]).[47,48] Fermented foods involve the action of lactic acid bacteria, acetic acid bacteria and propionic bacteria, and although they produce acid, these bacteria are unable to start a cavity.[49] If the bacteria are heated or destroyed in some way, the foods will only contain the acid by-products of the bacteria, but no bacteria. If, however, the foods are consumed with live bacteria, the foods will provide a good source of bacteria to out-produce and overtake cavity-causing bacteria. Due to the production of acid by these good bacteria, it is best to check your mouth pH after consumption, especially if you have poor buffering capacity. If you find that your mouth is acidic after eating these probiotic foods, don't stop eating them, just be aware that you need to manually neutralize your mouth after.

**How Often to Consume?**

The beneficial bacteria in yogurt has been found in the saliva of individuals up to three weeks after the consumption of yogurt was discontinued.[50] However other studies indicate that in order for recolonization of beneficial bacteria to occur in the mouth, there needs to be very frequent exposure to the probiotics.[51] Remember MS or cavity-causing bacteria are extremely resistant to being taken over or recolonized by new bacteria. The switch simply will not happen unless VERY high levels of the new bacteria are CONSISTENTLY present, and the existing MS bacteria are out-produced and starved.[52]

Ideally consume foods or probiotics containing cavity-resistant bacteria at every meal, especially at first during the initial recolonization period of time. At the bare minimum, consume probiotic foods once per day.

## 2. Probiotic Supplements

Probiotic capsules can be opened and emptied into a variety of foods and drinks to increase one's exposure to cavity-resistant bacteria. Make sure to check the ingredients, and do not use probiotics that contain ascorbic acid, or any potentially acidic or sugary additives.

- Open the capsule and empty it into a small amount of water. Swish the water and probiotic mixture in your mouth and swallow. Ideally leave it on your teeth for a while, for example, before going to bed or avoid drinking and eating for a period of time after.

- Open the capsule and carefully empty its contents onto your toothbrush bristles, with or without toothpaste.

- Empty the probiotics onto any foods and drinks that are not piping hot – remember that heat kills the bacteria.

## 3. Oral Probiotics

Probiotic chewing gum, lozenges.

## 4. Diet

GAPS (Gut and Psychology Syndrome) is a six-stage diet protocol designed to recolonize the body with good bacteria.[53]

## 5. Do Not Feed the Cavity-Causing Bacteria

Some studies have shown that cavity-resisting bacteria are only able to eliminate MS bacteria in the absence of sucrose.[54,55] Remember cavity-causing bacteria feed on sucrose.

# What About Lactobacilli?

Another group of bacteria that are associated with cavities are the lactobacilli. This is not a specific type or strain of bacteria, but rather a description of the shape of the bacteria (rod-shaped) under which an enormous number of bacteria fall into.[56] Some lactobacilli have been isolated from already-existing cavities, however current thinking is that lactobacilli are incapable of initiating or starting cavities, and can only contribute to the progression of an already-started cavity.[57] In other words, without the presence of MS bacteria, lactobacilli cannot cause a cavity. This is important to keep this in mind because many probiotics and probiotic foods contain lactobacilli.

I like to compare MS bacteria to a schoolyard bully. Just like the bacteria can start a cavity, the schoolyard bully can start a fight in the playground. The bully has friends who join in the fight, and before long the whole playground is in one giant fight with everyone pushing each other. But on the days when the bully stays home sick from school, the playground is peaceful and fun and everyone is playing with each other harmoniously. The bully's friends prefer to play fun games with everyone rather than fight, and so they happily join in the peaceful games. Absolutely no fighting is happening without the bully around, and the same occurs in the mouth – no cavities occur without the MS bacteria around. As soon as the bully returns to school, the fighting starts again. The bully's friends are like the lactobacilli bacteria. They won't start any trouble on their own, but they will join in the trouble once it has started. Lactobacilli may or may not contribute to problems, and it is dependent on whether MS bacteria have already started the cavity. They are like the kids in the schoolyard that really just want to play peacefully with the rest. They aren't the bully.

For example, in 2001, *Caries Research Journal* published a study that demonstrated the protective abilities of bacteria that fall into the classification of Lactobacilli. The study compared children who drank regular milk and those who drank milk with the addition of the bacteria, *Lactobacillus rhamnosus* GG. The children who drank the milk with bacteria had significantly lower levels of *Streptococcus mutans*, as well as significantly fewer cavities.[58]

## Testing for MS bacteria

How to know if you have MS/cavity-causing bacteria?

If you have active cavities, you have high levels of MS or cavity-causing bacteria. Although it is possible to prevent and remineralize cavities while maintaining a high level of these bacteria, it will definitely make it easier to do so by recolonizing with cavity-resistant bacteria.

If you have arrested cavities, and have not recolonized your mouth, you most likely still have a high level of MS or cavity-causing bacteria in your mouth. Good for you for arresting your decay! Without recolonizing your mouth bacteria, however, you will have to work harder to continue to keep your teeth free from future decay. If you recolonize your mouth with cavity-resisting bacteria, you will still obviously have to work at keeping your mouth healthy, but not nearly as hard because the good bacteria will be on your side, fighting off MS or cavity-causing bacteria every second of every day. All your efforts toward keeping a healthy mouth will be magnified in the presence of cavity-resisting bacteria.[59]

There are saliva tests available at your dentist's office to determine if you have a high number of *Streptococcus mutans* in your mouth. These tests are harmless, relatively inexpensive (you would have to inquire about exact pricing from your dentist's office) and tell you some very powerful information. I recommend getting tested at the following times, especially if you are susceptible to or have a history of cavities:

· Before or during pregnancy. If you have high levels of cavity-causing bacteria, you have the opportunity to reduce them so you can pass along cavity-resistant bacteria to your child. Some foods that contain cavity-resistant bacteria may not be acceptable to consume during pregnancy, so check with your healthcare provider first.

· Work at recolonizing your mouth for three to six months and then have your levels checked to monitor your progress. If you want to, you can have your *S. mutans* levels checked first, although it is quite likely you will test positive for high levels if you have or have had cavities and haven't recolonized your mouth. I would just assume that you have high levels.

Do not be disheartened if you are unable to recolonize your mouth. Lots of people have been able to be active-cavity-free while still maintaining a high level of MS bacteria – including myself.

Since we are unable to see the bacteria colonies within our mouth and on our teeth, we often underestimate the powerful impact they have upon our health. Indeed, the bacteria that have made a home on your teeth can either be your friends or your foe. Every single one of us has bacteria residing on our teeth. Encouraging the growth of cavity-resisting bacteria that will work hard to keep your teeth free from cavities at all times is a powerful way to keep your teeth protected.[60,61]

Unless you have made some purposeful and drastic changes in your mouth, the bacteria that colonized your teeth when they first appeared in your mouth, are usually the same bacteria found on your teeth throughout your entire life.[62] Of course, drastic changes can go the other way as well, and result in a changeover from non-pathogenic to pathogenic organisms. Overall health and function of the immune system has a significant role in one's microbial surveillance system and resistance to cavity-causing bacteria.[63] Focusing on natural prevention and remineralization methods will benefit oral health as well as overall health, and overall health will in turn positively affect oral health. What a lovely cycle to have occurring in one's body!

The Specific Plaque Hypothesis provides a powerful approach to protecting the teeth, however, I recommend employing aspects of both the Specific and Non-Specific Plaque Hypotheses in your prevention and remineralization strategy. This would involve the following:

· Ensuring as little bacteria as possible exist in the mouth at any given time (Non-Specific).

· Ensuring that the bacteria in the mouth are non-pathogenic and incapable of causing a cavity (Specific).

Instead of living in fear of cavity-causing bacteria, take control of your oral bacteria through both natural elimination strategies and recolonization, which will create the necessary environment for cavity prevention and remineralization.

# 6

# A Harsh or Helpful Environment: Saliva

"This 'drill and fill' approach was simply symptomatic treatment and failed to deal with the underlying etiologic factors."

*– Sturdevant's Art & Science of Operative Dentistry*[1]

At my office, I have a program for children who receive points when I see them with plaque-free teeth. They can save up their points for prizes. It is amazing how much this points program inspires children (and some adults!) to brush their teeth. Inspecting teeth for plaque has made me realize that some people develop loads and loads of plaque while others develop very little. Sometimes I see children and adults immediately after they brush their teeth, and they have more plaque on their teeth than some people who haven't brushed their teeth for hours! What are the two groups doing differently? How can the plaque-filled mouths become more like the perpetual plaque-free mouths?

Most often plaque contains acid-producing bacteria and when the plaque sits on a tooth, minerals are dissolved out. If you just focus on removing plaque with brushing and flossing, and do not focus on reducing the amount of plaque created in the first place, you are fighting an upward battle. Even though your teeth will be protected from the damaging effects of plaque immediately after brushings, shortly later plaque will return and your teeth will end up being in a harsh environment for much of the day. If you also focus on reducing the amount of plaque created in the first place, in between brushings your teeth will also be protected, and this is a more powerful and effective approach to take.

Saliva is the key to having perpetually low levels of plaque. Saliva is like the bodyguard for teeth and its job is to protect teeth from damage and to remineralize teeth after damage has occurred.

## Protective Functions of Saliva

· Forms the dental pellicle, which is a film that forms on the tooth to prevent against demineralization. The dental pellicle is a semi-permeable barrier that allows the remineralizing minerals, calcium and phosphate, to cross but not acids.[2]

· Self-Cleansing – imagine having a house that could clean itself. Well, that is what saliva does for our mouths! Saliva moves over our teeth and washes away plaque.

· Buffering Capacity – from bicarbonate and phosphate ions (see Chapter 4).

· Remineralization – saliva is designed to remineralize our teeth. Calcium and phosphate, the major minerals involved with remineralization are contained within the saliva.

· Antimicrobial – saliva contains important components that contribute to our immune system that are antifungal, antibacterial and antiviral.[3]

· Enzymes – digestion of food starts in mouth. Enzymes are important for helping clean the grooves in our teeth where food gets caught.

While saliva has an impressive job description, it simply cannot carry its functions out if we don't do *our* job and make sure we have enough saliva. The more saliva you have, the more your teeth are protected.

## Saliva Types

There are two types of saliva: Unstimulated and Stimulated. Unstimulated is also called 'Resting Saliva.' Unstimulated saliva refers to the saliva that is in the mouth while at rest – while the mouth is not eating or drinking anything. Not rest as in sitting versus working out, but rest for the mouth as in not chewing versus chewing or drinking. Talking does not count.

**Not Chewing Anything = Unstimulated/Resting Saliva**

Stimulated saliva refers to the saliva that is in the mouth while chewing something. Putting anything into your mouth triggers the brain to stimulate the flow of saliva through taste, muscle and esophageal receptors. Stimulated saliva always means *more* saliva is produced in the mouth.[4]

**Chewing Anything = Stimulated Saliva = More Saliva**

Stimulated saliva is not only more plentiful than unstimulated saliva but it contains less acid than unstimulated saliva. Stimulated saliva functions to protect the teeth from damage. Demineralization potential is highest during eating and right after because there is plenty of food for bacteria to consume and produce acid. The body attempts to protect teeth by producing lots of less-acidic saliva while food is in the mouth – stimulated saliva.

## How to Test Unstimulated/ Resting Saliva[5]

With one hand, roll your lower lip down to expose the wet inside part of your lip. Take a tissue and dry it off. Now start a timer and watch your lower lip very closely, still holding it rolled out. Watch for a tiny little droplet of saliva to appear on the inside part of your lip. As soon as you see a little droplet of saliva, check the timer to see how long it took. You will have to look very closely, otherwise you will miss seeing the tiny droplet of saliva.

### Results:

**0-30 seconds:** excellent amount of resting saliva

**31-45 seconds:** good/normal amount of resting saliva

**46-60 seconds:** low amount of resting saliva (risk for cavities)

**Over 60 seconds:** extremely low amount of resting saliva (high risk for cavities)

## How to Test Water Content in Saliva:[6]

Spit five times into a container and visually inspect the saliva.

### Visual Inspection of Collected Saliva:

**Clear and watery** = excellent level of water content

**Bubbly and stringy** = low water content (risk for cavities)

**Frothy and sticky** = very low water content (high risk for cavities)

# How to Test Stimulated Saliva[7]

Select something that is chewy, non-absorbent and will not fall apart when chewed. Suggestions are gum, honeycomb, paraffin wax or beeswax.

Obtain a milliliter measuring cup or milliliter syringe. These can be purchased at drug stores and even come free with some supplements and medications.

Set a timer for one minute and start chewing. As saliva pools in your mouth, **<u>do not swallow</u>**. Spit into the measuring cup or a regular cup if using a syringe to measure and continue chewing. Do not stop chewing; continue spitting as you feel the saliva pool in your mouth. If you do not feel saliva pool or do not feel like spitting, that is okay, just keep chewing and spit at the end of the one minute.

Stop chewing and spitting after one minute and measure the amount of saliva collected.

## Results:

**Greater than 5.0 ml** = Excellent

**3.5 ml - 5.0 ml** = Low (risk for cavities)

**Less than 3.5 ml** = Very Low (high risk for cavities)

(For added benefit, use pH paper to check the pH of the stimulated saliva. The ideal pH of stimulated saliva is neutral or alkaline. See Chapter 4.)

# Interpreting Your Results

Excellent or Good Resting Saliva

+ Excellent or Good Stimulated Saliva

+ Clear and Watery Saliva

= Congratulations!


Low or Extremely Low Resting Saliva
+ Excellent or Good Stimulated Saliva

= Dehydrated


Any Resting or Stimulated Saliva

+ Low or Very Low Water Content

= Dehydrated


Any level of Resting Saliva

+ Low or Extremely Low Stimulated Saliva

= Depleted Salivary Glands

# Natural Strategies to Increase Unstimulated and Stimulated Saliva Flow

If you are deficient in saliva, either unstimulated, stimulated or both, the steps to increase your production of saliva through natural methods is the same.

Unstimulated saliva can change drastically throughout the day, while stimulated saliva is much more constant. Improving your unstimulated saliva may be as simple as drinking more water, and your results could improve immediately. However, it could also be more complex, depending on the underlying source(s) of the deficiency. It may require some major lifestyle alterations and time. Generally speaking, improving unstimulated saliva will be easier and quicker to do than improving stimulated saliva. An analogy would be like improving a house by fixing a cracked tile on the floor (unstimulated saliva) and fixing a crack in the foundation or structural wall (stimulated saliva). Even though the larger crack will require more work and time, repairing both is very important.

## Address the Following:

### 1. Mouth Breathing

Mouth breathing will result in a dry mouth and an increased risk of cavities, as well as gum disease and other systemic concerns. As previously discussed, mouth breathing can induce some undesirable dental and systemic issues. Although likely challenging and time-consuming, addressing the cause(s) of mouth breathing will be worthwhile.

Until I made some diet and lifestyle changes, I used to be a mouth breather every summer with seasonal allergies, and will still occasionally catch myself mouth breathing if I eat certain foods. Every summer my teeth felt gross with increased plaque, and I even noticed that food tasted slightly different and duller. Now I have teeth that are cleaner than when I was a mouth breather – even when I don't brush my teeth.

## 2. Drink More Water

Most people know they should be drinking an adequate amount of water, but perhaps undervalue its importance when it comes to oral health.

Water Filtration Systems

Many people have water filters of varying types, and while it is good to drink water free of toxins, sometimes water can also have all of its minerals removed. Drinking water that is devoid of minerals and not somehow replacing those minerals in your body will lead to oral and overall health concerns.

For example, distilled water contains no minerals. Studies have demonstrated that when a tooth is placed in distilled water that has a neutral (not acidic) pH, small amounts of minerals dissolve out of the tooth because the water contains no calcium or phosphate.[8] Even though the water is not acidic, minerals still dissolve away because of the concentration gradient or difference between the minerals in the water and in the tooth.

I encourage you to find a source of water and/or filter that you are happy with that contains plenty of minerals and no or few toxins. And drink more of it!

## 3. Medications

Drugs are considered to be the most common cause of decreased saliva. It is thought that hundreds and possibly thousands of drugs are capable of negatively affecting saliva output.[9] People who are taking medications for hypertension, depression and other psychiatric illnesses, allergies and urinary conditions are most at risk for having depleted salivary output as a side effect of the drugs.[10,11]

## 4. Stress

Saliva production is significantly slowed during times of stress. Remember, saliva is not something that will help the body during an emergency situation, so production is reduced until a later time when the body returns to a more relaxed state. Chronic stress is associated with deficient saliva output.[12,13]

## 5. Smoking[14]

## 6. Recreational Drug Use[15]

7. **Caffeine**, such as coffee, tea, soft drinks and energy drinks.[16]

## 8. Alcohol[17]

(If you have extremely low salivary function it would be best to even avoid alcohol-containing mouthwash.)[18]

### 9. Hormonal Imbalance

Saliva production and composition is partially regulated by hormones. Alterations in hormone levels, especially estrogen is associated with decreased production of both types of saliva, as well as changes in composition. [19,20,21]

### 10. Food

Food plays a significant role in helping or hindering saliva reduce the creation of plaque. Different foods will result in more or less plaque formation. Sugary foods result in increased plaque formation. This includes refined sugars and unrefined sugars. Unrefined sugars offer great benefits over refined, such as the inclusion of vitamins and minerals that refined sugars are lacking. However, reduced dental plaque formation is not one of the benefits of unrefined sugars – indeed, both refined and unrefined sugars will feed bacteria and lead to increased accumulation of plaque. Consuming cooked starches is also associated with increased plaque accumulation, and raw starches are associated with decreased plaque accumulation.[22]

Often people who have a dry mouth will suck on candies or chew gum to increase saliva in their mouth. This is because candies and gum induce stimulated saliva production, which is more plentiful than unstimulated. However, many times candies and gum contain sugar, and if they are sugar-free, can be highly acidic. The stimulated saliva will help protect teeth while the candy or gum is in the mouth, but once the person stops chewing and returns to a resting state of deficient saliva, the sugar or acid can cause some significant damage to the teeth. Check your mouth pH during and after using any product, and ideally address the underlying issue of having a dry mouth so that you do not have to rely on products, and can use them as treats instead. Sucking on ice cubes (not chewing) might be a good alternative for some people.[23]

## Important but Overlooked

Saliva, often overlooked and undervalued, plays a significant role in determining whether the tooth environment is helpful or harsh. Knowing where one stands with regards to the details of saliva production provides insight into a powerful aspect of cavity prevention and remineralization.

# 7

# A Strong or Susceptible Tooth: MMPs

"The patient's general health has a significant impact on overall caries risk."

– *Sturdevant's Art & Science of Operative Dentistry.*[1]

Picture a beautiful garden full of flowers. The flowers are all healthy and every petal in perfect bloom. In order to keep the garden in such great condition, the gardener tends to it every day. When flowers die, the gardener trims them off. The gardener knows that removing the dead flowers will allow for new healthy flowers to grow even better.

Matrix metalloproteinases are like the gardener in our body. When tissues are damaged or die, matrix metalloproteinases trim off the dead or damaged parts so that new, healthy tissues can grow.

Matrix metalloproteinases (MMPs) are a group of enzymes responsible for breaking down or destroying proteins, such as collagen, gelatin and proteoglycans, which are found in skin, bones, connective tissue and teeth.[2] While it may seem like MMPs are bad because they are destroying body parts, they are, in fact, essential. Just like trimming off the dead flowers on a plant so new ones can grow better, MMPs remove parts of the body that have been damaged so that healing can take place. When damage has occurred somewhere in the body, MMPs are released and activated. The damaged tissue is then broken down and destroyed by the MMPs, so that new healthy tissue can be laid down to replace the damaged. MMPs are an important part of the healing process.

**MMP = Matrix Metalloproteinase**

**MMP = enzyme that breaks down damaged body parts**

(Matrix Metalloproteinases are also sometimes called Matrixins.)[3]

But what if the gardener doesn't stop picking even after all the dead flowers have been removed? Instead, the gardener continues picking off the flowers in bloom, the leaves, the stems...and soon what used to be a healthy plant is now destroyed. What started off as a healthy act for the plant, trimming dead flowers off, didn't stop and actually caused so much damage that the plant was destroyed. Just like the gardener needs to stop picking after all the dead flowers have been removed to avoid further destruction, so too do MMPs need to be deactivated after all the damaged tissue has been removed. Without deactivation, MMPs will continue breaking down tissue, moving on to healthy tissue, resulting in damage. What started out as a healthy, healing process can became a very unhealthy, destructive process.

Deactivators of MMPs are called matrix metalloproteinase inhibitors, of which TIMPs are the most prevalent.

**TIMP = Tissue Inhibitor Metalloproteinase**

TIMPs are proteins that form complexes with MMPs and render them inactive.[4] Matrix metalloproteinase inhibitors such as TIMPs, are like the gardener's boss who tells the gardener to stop working. TIMPs maintain a balance between essential degradation, allowing for healthy regeneration and excessive degradation, resulting in damage.

Damage occurs when there is too much MMP production and/or too little TIMPs to deactivate the MMPs.[5]

**MMPs balanced by TIMPs**
**= Damaged tissues removed so that new tissue can grow**
**= Healthy healing**

**Excessive MMPs + Insufficient TIMPs**
**= Damaged tissues *and* healthy tissues removed**
**= Destruction**

For example, when a wound occurs on the skin, MMPs are synthesized by both the wounded skin cells and inflammatory cells. The MMPs destroy the damaged skin by breaking it apart, and continue to destroy tissue until deactivated by TIMPs. Non-healing wounds have a higher number of MMPs and a lower number of TIMPs. Too many MMPs and not enough inhibitors of MMPs to stop their action, results in continued damage and a lack of healing.[6]

Matrix metalloproteinases (MMPs) are involved with nearly all tissues of the body in both normal functioning and pathological events. MMPs are critical for cell growth and survival, host defence systems, tissue remodeling and development. This includes teeth and cavities.[7]

## MMPs & Cavities

MMPs are synthesized and secreted by connective tissue cells, including odontoblasts, and are found in both saliva and teeth.[8,9,10,11]

In teeth, MMPs function to keep teeth healthy. Bacterial acids cause demineralization and the dissolution of hydroxyapatite – minerals are removed. This is damage that requires MMPs to clean up. The bacterial acids and demineralization is like a flower dying. MMPs are synthesized and activated and proceed to digest the demineralized, damaged dentin, and the damaged tooth tissue is removed. Damaged dentin and enamel[12] are cleaned up to allow for tissue remodeling, regeneration and healing.[13] MMPs stimulate growth factors necessary for reparative dentin formation, the dentin that is produced in response to cavities in an attempt to slow the rate of progression and remineralize the tooth.[14,15] The highest ratio of MMPs to TIMPs is found at the junction of enamel and dentin, called the dentinoenamel junction (DEJ). This is why a cavity significantly spreads laterally once it extends through the enamel and reaches the dentin,[16] giving dentin cavities their characteristic triangle shape, with the wide base facing out, at the DEJ, and the pointed triangle tip deep into dentin, towards the pulp.[17]

MMPs determine how fast dentin is degraded.[18] Like the gardener with no boss around to stop him, he will continue cutting out all the flowers and destroy the garden. When there are lots of MMPs around and few TIMPs to inactivate them, the damaged dentin will be removed, as well as the healthy dentin. This is a situation in which the cavity progresses. A healthy balance of MMPs and TIMPs however, will result in just the damaged dentin being removed so that healthy dentin can replace it, and the healing process sets in. TIMPs act like the boss, stopping the progression of a cavity.

**MMPs balanced by TIMPs**
**= Damage caused by bacterial acids removed**
**= Healthy healing of tooth and cavity**

**Excessive MMPs + Insufficient TIMPs**
**= Damaged caused by bacterial acids *and* healthy dentin removed**
**= Cavity progression**

# Developing Teeth

MMPs play a major role in developing teeth and the production of dentin, called dentinogenesis.[19,20] You can give your child an amazing life-long gift; the gift of strong, healthy teeth that will resist cavities for the rest of their life. An important way to give them this gift is by ensuring they have an ideal balance of MMPs and TIMPs so that their teeth develop optimally.

# Bacterial or Human?

Bacteria also have matrix metalloproteinases. It used to be thought that the bacterial MMPs were responsible for the destruction of dentin. However, more recent research does not support that idea.[21,22,23,24]

In 1998, the *Journal of Dental Research* published a study of a joint effort between researchers at the University of British Columbia and the University of Helsinki.

The study looked at which enzymes were responsible for the destruction of dentin during the progression of a cavity. (Remember a cavity starts with demineralization or the removal of minerals from enamel, and then progresses to the inside part of the tooth which is dentin.)

The researchers exposed some demineralized dentin to cavity-causing bacterial MMPs and some demineralized dentin to sterilized human MMPs, containing no bacteria. Only the dentin exposed to human MMPs resulted in further degradation or progression of the cavity. The dentin exposed to the bacterial MMPs did not have any activity or breakdown at all.[25]

**Dentin in acid + Human MMPs = cavity progression**

**Dentin in acid + Bacterial MMPs**

**= no further progression**

What does this mean?

After bacteria initiate a cavity in enamel, the progression of the cavity is caused by the person's own MMPs.[26,27]

Imagine someone is at a picnic. It is a beautiful day, the sun is shining, the kids are playing together peacefully and the food the person prepared is a delicious hit with everyone. Several bees are flying around the food and the person laughs and says, "Oh no bees, this is our tasty food," and calmly covers the food up with some picnic nets. What a wonderful day.

Imagine another scene. Same person out at a picnic. But this day is rainy and cold. The kids are fighting and screaming at each other. The food is soggy from the rain and doesn't taste very good. And then come the bees. The person angrily swats away at the bees and accidentally knocks over the dessert onto the muddy ground. Mumbling some not-so-nice words, the person picks up the ruined dessert while a bee is flying around it. Swatting at the bee again, it stings the person. Not a wonderful day.

While it may seem like the bees are responsible for the bad situation, upon closer inspection, one realizes that it cannot be the bees. The bees were the same in both situations, but the outcomes were significantly different. The outcomes were not dependent on the bees, but rather the circumstances at the picnic. Similarly, while it may seem like bacteria are responsible for the progression of a cavity, the reality is that it is the circumstances within the body that determines the extent of the damage of the cavity.

Like the bees, cavity-causing bacteria are an irritant. The cavity-causing bacteria initiate a cavity within the enamel of a tooth (the outer shell). MMPs are released to clean up the damaged tissue so that healing can take place. When MMPs are balanced by TIMPs, it is like the first picnic scenario where there are bees present but the damage caused by them is minimal. However, when there is a surplus of MMPs and a deficiency of MMP inhibitors in the body, it is like the rainy picnic with ruined food and fighting children. The MMPs that were originally released to clean up the damage caused by the cavity-causing bacteria are not deactivated and continue causing damage, resulting in the progression of the cavity through dentin.

So how does one have a sunny-day picnic instead of a rainy-day picnic in their body? How does one figuratively put the picnic nets over their food and enjoy the day, the equivalent of MMPs being deactivated after clearing damage from cavity-causing bacteria? And how does one make sure they do not end up swatting at bees, knocking over the dessert and getting stung – the equivalent of MMPs not being deactivated and continual destruction of dentin resulting in a progressing cavity?

A balance between MMPs and TIMPs (or MMP inhibitors) is essential for teeth to function properly (and the rest of the body). When one or the other is out of balance, cavities will develop and progress.[28]

**Excessive MMPs = Cavity progresses**

**Insufficient TIMPs or MMP Inhibitors**

**= Cavity progresses**

# How to Achieve Optimal MMPs and TIMPs

## 1. Neutral pH

Acidic pH levels have been shown to directly lead to activation of MMPs, when otherwise they would not be activated.[29,30,31] (See Chapter 4 for more information about maintaining a neutral mouth.)

# 2. MMP Inhibitors
# For Systemic Use

Tissue breakdown by MMPs has been shown to be a precursor for cancer cell invasion, metastasis or the spreading of cancer cells and for angiogenesis.[32] Synthetic MMP inhibitor drugs have been used to treat cancer since the 1990s, and over the years better drugs have been developed that are more effective and with fewer side effects.[33,34,35,36,37]

The presence of MMPs in the blood is also considered to be an early sign of heart damage, and MMP inhibitors are being used as a novel approach to heart damage prevention.[38]

## MMP Inhibitors for Dentistry

These MMP inhibitor drugs, while important for other diseases, are inappropriate for use to treat oral conditions, such as cavities, due to their side effects.[39] There is, however, currently a TIMP drug approved for use in dentistry, to treat gum disease (periodontal disease). Periostat, or low dose doxycycline, is a matrix metalloproteinase inhibitor. Gum disease is now known to have a very similar pattern with MMPs as cavities do. Damage caused by bacterial toxins – from bacteria associated with gum disease – initiates the person's own MMPs to clear the damaged tissue. Excessive MMP activity results in the breakdown of healthy tissues – gums, connective tissue and bone – and the progression of gum disease.

Another MMP inhibitor is used today in dentistry. Chlorhexidine is an antimicrobial agent commonly used as a mouthrinse or topical gel for the treatment of gum disease and cavities. Chlorhexidine is often used to treat bacterial infection, however studies have also shown that it is an effective MMP inhibitor.[40]

MMP inhibitors, the majority of which are TIMPS, have been shown to reduce cavity progression.[41,42] MMP inhibitors have also been shown to increase the longevity of bonded dental restorations by preventing recurrent decay at the margins.[43,44,45]

## Natural MMP Inhibitors

The following is a list of natural substances that have been shown to have MMP inhibition abilities:

· Avocado. Avocado has been shown to be effective at reducing MMP levels, including within the mouth. [46]

· *Lupinus albus* seeds. Commonly known as lupin or lupini beans, these are a popular snack in the Mediterranean. Normally lupini beans are soaked in sea water and consumed raw.[47] Lupini beans have the ability to reduce the levels of MMPs in inflamed tissues of the mouth.[48]

· Oleic acid. Oleic acid, the predominant fat in olive oil[49], has been shown to reduce MMPs.[50,51]

· Green tea. Green tea polyphenols have been shown to be potent inhibitors of MMP activation.[52,53,54,55]

## 3. Mercury

Mercury compounds can activate inactive MMPs. In other words, even when there is no damage and no job for MMPs to do, in the presence of mercury compounds, MMPs will be activated.[56] Selenium offsets damage incurred by mercury, so I strongly suggest obtaining optimal levels of selenium.[57]

### Sources of Selenium:[58]

- Garlic

- Onions

- Broccoli

- Egg Yolk

- Red Grapes

- Brazil Nuts

## 4. Oxidative Stress

Oxidative stress occurs when free radicals are not balanced with antioxidants. To understand how to minimize oxidative stress, it is first necessary to know what free radicals and antioxidants are.

# Free Radicals & Antioxidants

Imagine the following scene: it's cold outside, in fact it's winter in Canada. Even though it is cold, the molecule "people" are happy because they are walking around all bundled up. They have nice warm jackets and cozy hats and mittens. Being warm and happy, they calmly walk around and interact nicely with each other. But uh oh, here comes the free radical. The free radical is freezing cold because it doesn't have any clothes on. The free radical is so incredibly cold that it runs around like a lunatic trying to grab clothes off the happy and warmly clothed molecules. In the body, instead of missing clothing, free radicals are missing an electron. Missing an electron makes the molecule incredibly unstable and desperate to steal an electron from a nearby happy molecule. The process of trying to steal an electron from another molecule results in damage to the previously happy molecule, or even creates another free radical. Picture the crazy, naked free radical running around ripping clothing off the once-happy molecules. Their jackets get torn, they lose mittens and their toques are ripped off their heads. The free radical has a toque on its head, one mitten on and a handful of torn jacket pieces. The free radical is still naked and freezing cold, desperately running around, but now the molecules that were previously warm and happy are really cold and miserable. The miserable molecules start running around desperately trying to steal clothes from other happy, warmly clothed molecules. More and more damage occurs. The regular molecules do not have a spare electron to give to a free radical, just like the happy, warmly clothed people don't have spare clothes to give away. Even though the free radical tries to get an electron, there simply is not a spare electron to take, and the end result is just more and more damage.

But oh, here comes the antioxidant! The antioxidant is all bundled up with a warm snowsuit, scarf, hat and gloves, and look what it's carrying! Shopping bags! Full of warm clothing. The antioxidant finds the free radical, pulls warm clothes out of the shopping bags and dresses the free radical. Nice warm socks and boots, a track suit and warm coat, hat and gloves. The antioxidant is not damaged and doesn't lose any of its own clothing because it had extra clothing to donate to the free radical. And the free radical is no longer a free radical, but a happy, warm and calm molecule. It is no longer frantically running around causing damage. In come a few more antioxidants with hands full of shopping bags. They patch up the damaged molecules that had their clothing ripped by the free radical, replace their missing mittens or toques and give them new jackets. The molecules that had become free radicals stop running around frantically causing damage and are no longer free radicals. All is well now! In the body, antioxidants have an extra electron that they easily donate to free radicals missing them. Donating the electron does not damage the antioxidant, unlike regular molecules that are damaged in the presence of free radicals.

## Free Radicals & Matrix Metalloproteinases

The mitochondria is the part of a cell where energy is made. Energy is called ATP (adenosine triphosphate). Energy production is a highly important process, and the process during which energy is produced involves several steps within the mitochondria. One of the final steps results in an oxygen molecule that is missing an electron (called a reactive oxygen species, or more generally, a free radical). This is a highly unstable and rather dangerous molecule. Oxidative stress refers to free radical creation from energy production. I know I paint a bad picture of free radicals, but they are actually a part of healthy functioning. Just living and breathing and producing energy creates free radicals – so don't try to stop producing free radicals! You may be wondering why on earth our bodies produce free radicals, since they seem so dangerous and harmful. Free radicals actually are very important for the proper functioning of the body. Free radicals are messengers sending signals to modulate how cells function. They are able to activate enzymes and other processes in the body through a signaling process. This signaling is called, 'redox signaling,' because antioxidants cause *re*-duction and free radicals cause *ox*-idation.

Reduction is the when an electron is donated and oxidation is when an electron is lost.

## Redox Signaling & Cavities

Redox signaling is responsible for signaling the need to activate MMPs.[59,60,61] In other words, free radicals activate MMPs.

### Free Radicals → Activate MMPs

Naturally occurring free radicals – the ones produced from energy production – are supposed to be used to activate MMPs. However, free radicals from outside sources can also lead to the activation of MMPs because they use up antioxidants, leading to an excess of the naturally produced free radicals.[62,63,64]

Let's pretend you have five naturally produced free radicals and five antioxidants to balance them. The result is healthy and normal signaling of MMP activation. Now let's pretend that in addition to the five naturally produced free radicals, you also have five free radicals from outside sources. The five antioxidants are used to balance out the five new free radicals, and there are now five naturally produced free radicals left. These free radicals proceed to do their normal job and signal pathways in the body to produce MMPs, and the MMPs do their normal job and break down tissue, connective tissue, bone and dentin in teeth. Even though these molecules are all doing their normal job, the result is increased damage (including cavity progression) because of the excess of free radicals.

Another way that increased damage can occur is if there are insufficient antioxidants. Let's say you have five naturally produced free radicals and two antioxidants. The excess free radicals will proceed to signal for increased MMP activation, which in turns leads to cavity progression.

What about if you have five naturally produced free radicals, five free radicals from outside sources and only two antioxidants?... Imagine the extent of damage that would occur.

Thus, both naturally occurring free radicals and free radicals from outside sources can increase levels of MMPs, and contribute to cavity progression. Antioxidants can behave as MMP inhibitors by reducing the numbers of free radicals, and protect the tooth and cavity from continued damage.

↑ **Free Radicals = Cavity progression**

**Antioxidants = Protect tooth from excessive damage**

A strategic goal for reducing MMP damage and cavity progression is to decrease free radicals and increase antioxidants.

# Sources of Free Radicals:

· **Smoking.**[65] Did you know that children exposed to second-hand smoke have more cavities?[66]

· **Xenobiotics,**[67] are substances that are foreign to the body – such as pesticides and pollutants.[68]

· **Ionizing Radiation**[69]

· **Stress**[70]

· **Nutritional Deficiency.** Nutritional deficiency indirectly increases free radicals because many nutrients are necessary for the proper functioning of naturally produced antioxidants within the body. For example, zinc, copper and manganese are required for the naturally produced antioxidant, superoxide dismutase, and selenium is required for the naturally produced antioxidant glutathione peroxidase.[71] Magnesium deficiency is also associated with increased oxidative stress.[72]

· **Alcohol.**[73] Remember not to mix alcohol with acetaminophen. This creates potent free radicals which deplete the body of the antioxidant, glutathione.[74,75]

· **_Excessive_ Exercise.** Exercise is a source of oxidative stress. Remember oxidative stress is normal and healthy, and should occur in normal and healthy individuals. However, it needs to be balanced with antioxidants.[76]

## Sources of Antioxidants:

An antioxidant is any substance that can neutralize free radicals or their actions.[77] Antioxidants are produced within our body and are also obtained from food sources.

Antioxidants are commonly found in: [78]

- **Fruits**

- **Vegetables**

- **Supplements**

- **Spices**

- **Herbs**

There are many natural sources of antioxidants. I recommend looking at the ORAC (Oxygen radical absorbance capacity) values for foods and natural products online, and/or speaking with a nutritionist or dietician.

## Grapes to Remineralize Teeth?

Grape seed extract contains a high level of proanthocyanidin. Proanthocyanidin is an antioxidant and free radical scavenger that is found in some plants. Proanthocyanidin is part of a large group of plant antioxidants called polyphenols. In 2012, *The Journal of Contemporary Dental Practice* published a study detailing an experiment where grape seed extract was used as a remineralizing agent for extracted human teeth in which cavities were induced. Not only did the grape seed extract successfully remineralize the cavities, but it actually outperformed the other known remineralizing agents that were used as controls in the experiment.[79]

In addition to its antioxidant effects, proanthocyanidin is thought to be able to remineralize cavities by increasing collagen cross-links, which effectively make teeth stronger.[80]

## How to Know Your Oxidative Stress Levels?

There are a variety of tests available for testing your level of oxidative stress and/or antioxidant levels. Speak to your healthcare provider if you are interested in testing.

## Connecting it All Together

Matrix metalloproteinases provide an explanation for the incredibly intimate relationship between cavity-causing bacteria and the ensuing response that follows within the individual. Bacteria are the initial irritant, and the extent of destruction or progression of cavity is determined by the individual. MMPs also provide some idea for the drastic variation in cavity progression from one individual to the next. Perhaps as the connection that MMPs have with cavities becomes more well-known there will be new generations of children with strong teeth that are protected from cavities.

# 8

# A Strong or Susceptible Tooth: Hormones

"As in any other organ with a number of biologic activities, different malfunctions can occur which adversely affect the health of the tooth. The problems are not amenable to one simple solution. Life is complex whether it concerns a tooth or the whole body."

*– Dentinal Fluid Transport*[1]

My husband was driving and I was in the passenger seat. I pulled down the mirror in front of me and checked to make sure my makeup was not smudged and I had no food in my teeth. All good. Except that I caught a little glimpse of something different on the biting surface (occlusal) of one of my lower molars. "Weird," I thought, and made a mental note to check it out in detail at my dental office.

"I have a little cavity!" Initially I was really shocked. I had never had a cavity before. But after a brief moment of panic, I talked myself into looking at the bright side. I had an opportunity to practice what I preach. I always say that cavities are an awesome opportunity to learn that the body needs some TLC or improvement in some way.

It took me a little time, but once I figured out what needed improvement in my body, the small cavity hardened up. I felt so much better and noticed an improvement in my overall health! Even though I was eating a very nutritious diet, I was not feeling at the peak of my health, and it is really no surprise that I got a cavity at that time of my life. It was time for me to learn about hormones, both overall and how they affect oral health.

Of course, all hormones and hormonal systems are important aspects of cavity prevention. Remember overall health impacts oral health, and if any hormones are not functioning optimally, oral health can be negatively affected.[2] However, there are two specific hormones that have been directly linked with cavities and I will discuss these in detail:

Thyroid Hormones

Estrogen

# Thyroid

## Thyroid Function & Cavities

Studies have shown that cavities are inversely related to thyroid function. That is, as thyroid function decreases, incidence of cavities increases.[3,4,5,6,7,8,9] Given that thyroid disorders are on the rise, especially among women,[10,11] optimizing thyroid health is essential for natural prevention and remineralization of cavities. It is estimated that over 12 million Americans have thyroid dysfunction with 60% of these people not even aware of it.[12]

The thyroid gland is located on the trachea (the throat), and is responsible for the production and secretion of the vital hormones, triiodothyronine (called T3) and thyroxine (called T4). Hypothyroidism is an underactive thyroid, and is associated with an increased risk of cavities (see above references 2-8).

# How Does Low Thyroid Increase Cavities?

Hormones are small molecules that can produce some major physiological changes in the body. Hormones do not bind to every cell in the body, but rather specific tissues that are designed to bind to the hormones. These specific tissues have what are called target cells. Target cells contain receptors that bind to the hormone. It is like the hormone is walking around a parking lot with a key trying to find the car that fits. Most cars do not fit the key, but once it finds the right car and turns the lock, it can open the door, start the car and drive away. Same within the body, when the hormone finds its target cell with the receptor that fits the hormone perfectly, the target cell then proceeds to carry out the necessary physiological functions that the hormone is designed to do.

## Hormone → Target Cell with Receptor

## → Physiological Changes Occur[13]

This is how the thyroid and cavities are related. Thyroid hormones T3 and T4 are produced in the thyroid gland, and are then transported by the blood to tissues located throughout the entire body. The salivary glands contain target cells that have receptors for the thyroid hormones. Once bound to the hormones, the target cells initiate a chain reaction of events that result in the production of saliva that is protective to teeth. The saliva produced when plenty of thyroid hormone is bound to the salivary glands is less acidic and contains more protein.

When there is little hormone present to bind to the target cell receptors, the physiological functions that are supposed to be carried out do not occur, or they occur in an altered manner.

## ~~Hormone~~ → Target Cell with Receptor

## → ~~Physiological Changes Occur~~

Similarly, when there is deficiency of thyroid hormones, the target cells within the salivary glands are not able to carry out the functions they are designed to do. As a result, saliva is still produced, but is less protective to teeth. It is more acidic and contains less protein.[14] More acidic saliva puts the tooth at higher risk of demineralization; less protein in the saliva can lower buffering abilities.[15]

I had always had consistently neutral saliva, and even though I frequently talked about pH testing to people, I hadn't actually tested my own saliva for a couple of years. However, after I noticed the little cavity on my tooth, I started testing my saliva pH again and was shocked to learn it had become consistently acidic!

## Calcitonin

In addition to T3 and T4 hormones, the thyroid also produces calcitonin, a hormone that controls calcium metabolism, along with the parathyroid hormone. The parathyroid hormone (produced by the parathyroid gland) mobilizes calcium from bones and teeth when blood-calcium levels are low. Calcitonin is responsible for calcium being deposited into bones and teeth when blood-calcium levels are adequate or high. Thus, calcitonin slows down the breakdown of bone and teeth, and this can be impaired by decreased thyroid function.[16,17]

# Symptoms of Hypothyroidism[18]

- Weight gain
- Low body temperature
- Inability to tolerate cold
- Sparse, coarse, dry hair
- Coarse, dry, scaly, thick skin
- Yellowish appearance on the hands and feet
- Thinning outer edge of eyebrows
- Confusion, forgetfulness
- Low iron levels
- Hoarse voice
- Slowed speech
- Dull facial expression
- Droopy eyelids
- Puffy face and eyes
- Carpal tunnel syndrome

# Hashimoto's Thyroiditis

Hashimoto's thyroiditis, an autoimmune disorder, is considered to be the most common cause of hypothyroidism. An autoimmune disorder occurs when the body attacks itself, and in the case of Hashimoto's thyroiditis, inflammation and damage occurs to the thyroid gland.[19]

# Risk Factors for Thyroid Dysfunction

## 1. C-reactive Protein

C-reactive protein is a blood marker of inflammation. It is a simple blood test and will give you an indication of the level of inflammation in your body. Studies have shown that both mild to severe hypothyroidism is associated with elevated C-reactive protein.[20] Talk to your healthcare provider about being tested for it.

(High levels of C-reactive protein are also associated with gum disease.)[21,22,23,24]

## 2. Estrogen

Excessive levels of estrogen can impair thyroid functioning.[25]

## 3. Iodine Deficiency

Centers for Disease Control and Prevention (CDC) considers iodine deficiency one of the major deficiency diseases in the world.[26] Iodine deficiency does not just affect developing countries and, in fact, the incidence of iodine deficiency has risen significantly in the United States, with women of child-bearing age and pregnant women most at risk.[27,28]

Iodine is not a hormone, but like hormones, iodine has specific receptors on target cells to which it binds, initiating a chain reaction to occur so that physiological functions can be carried out. The receptors for iodine are called sodium iodide (Na+/I) symporters and require sodium and iodine together in order to cause a physiological response.[29]

It is commonly known that iodine is necessary for proper functioning of the thyroid gland. This means that the thyroid gland contains target cells with sodium-iodide symporters so that iodine can bind to them. Iodine is also necessary for proper functioning of the salivary glands, meaning there are target cells with sodium-iodide symporters within the salivary glands.[30,31] When there is not enough iodine in the salivary glands to bind to the target cells, the result is a deficiency of saliva production.

**Impaired Thyroid Function = Acidic Saliva**

**Low Iodine = Less Saliva (Dry Mouth)**

**Low Iodine → Impaired Thyroid Function**

**= Acidic Saliva + Less Saliva = High Risk of Cavities**

## Other Iodine Receptors:

In addition to salivary glands and the thyroid, iodine receptors have also been found in the following tissues: [32,33]

- Pancreas
- Heart
- Lacrimal glands (eyes)
- Adrenal gland
- Pituitary gland
- Testes
- Choroid pluxes (spine)
- Mammary glands (breasts)
- Ovaries
- Prostate
- Gastric mucosa
- Thymus
- Lung

Iodine deficiency is related to stillbirth, spontaneous abortion and reduced intellectual development in babies.[34]

## Too Much Iodine

Extremes one way or the other are not healthy, and iodine is no exception. Too little or too much iodine is not ideal. Paradoxically, like inadequate amounts of iodine, too much iodine can also lead to thyroid dysfunction.[35] However, the fear of too much iodine should not prevent someone and/or healthcare practitioners from ensuring that enough iodine is being obtained.[36] "Without trivializing its seriousness, most observers agree that the risk of iodine-induced hyperthyroidism should not obscure the many benefits that iodine has for women and children, and should not slow the pace toward proper correction of the deficiency in a community."[37]

## How to Ensure Adequate Iodine Levels:

### Iodine Food Sources:

· Products of the sea:[38]

  - Sea vegetables, such as kelp

  - Seafoods, such as sardines, shellfish, fish

  - Salt

· Multivitamins. Some multivitamins contain iodine.

· Iodine Supplements. Too much iodine can be harmful, which can occur with iodine supplementation. You must be under the care of a healthcare practitioner if you are considering supplementation.

### Limit Bromine Exposure

Iodine, fluorine, bromine, chlorine and astatine all belong to the same group of elements called halogens. Halogens share similar properties and are also similarly shaped. Iodine receptors, which are supposed to bind to iodine, have been shown to also bind to bromine.[39,40,41] When bromine binds to iodine receptors, the physiological functions that are supposed to be carried out by iodine do not occur. Functioning of the tissues containing iodine receptors, such as salivary glands and thyroid are impaired when iodine is not able to bind to the receptors due to competition.[42]

**Iodine + Iodine Receptors**

**= Optimal Functioning of Salivary Glands and Thyroid (and other tissues)**

**Iodine + Bromine + Iodine Receptors**

**= ~~Iodine~~ + Bromine = Lack of Optimal Functioning**

Imagine someone already has iodine deficiency. In the presence of bromine, iodine deficiency is magnified, because of the competition with bromine.

## Bromine Sources

Common bromine sources include:

## 1. Bleaching Agent[43]

Bromine is used as a bleaching agent in flour (both white and whole wheat).

## 2. Cleaning products

Bromine can be absorbed through the skin as well as through inhalation.[44]

## 3. Disinfectant[45]

Bromine is found in swimming pools and hot tubs.

## 4. Pesticides[46]

## 5. Soft Drinks

Bromine is added to vegetable oil and used as an emulsifier to prevent separation in citrus soft drinks, and is called BVO (brominated vegetable oil). BVO as a food additive is banned in some parts of the world, such as Europe and Australia, but is approved for use in North America. Due to pressure from online petitions, Coca-Cola and Pepsi have agreed to stop using BVO in their products such as Powerade, Gatorade and Mountain Dew. As of May 5, 2014, Coca-Cola and Pepsi no longer use BVO in their soft drinks, although it is still approved for use in North America. Generic brands of citrus sodas and other companies still use BVO. BVO was replaced with sucrose acetate isobutyrate, a food additive that is generally regarded as safe, which is what BVO is also considered to be.[47,48] I recommend avoiding soft drinks, regardless of whether they contain BVO or not.

## 6. Flame Retardants[49]

Organobromide is a flame retardant used in mattresses.

## See Your HealthCare Provider

If you have been diagnosed with thyroid dysfunction or suspect that you might have issues with your thyroid, please speak with your healthcare practitioner about ways to naturally and/or synthetically improve your thyroid functioning. An in-depth discussion about improving thyroid function is beyond the scope of this book and my expertise as a dentist.

Thyroid dysfunction does not mean a life full of cavities. Being aware of a potential increased susceptibility to cavities helps you be prepared and take action to protect your teeth, making your dreams of a cavity-free mouth come true.

# Estrogen

# Women & Cavities

Since the agricultural revolution, there is documentation that females have been experiencing, on average, slightly higher rates of cavities than men.[50,51] The trend has continued throughout the nineteenth and twentieth centuries, and today recent meta-analysis studies of countries worldwide indicate similar findings.[52]

The following statistics are from the National Institute of Dental and Craniofacial Research of data collected in the United States between 1994 and 2004:[53]

· 2.09% more females have cavities than men (although very high numbers of both genders have cavities – over 90%).

· Females have greater DMFT numbers than men. DMFT is the number of decayed, missing, and filled teeth. This gives an indication of the severity of the cavities. On average, females have 10.70 decayed, missing or filled teeth while men have on average 9.95 decayed, missing or filled teeth.

## Estrogen & Cavities

Estrogen has been shown to cause an increase in cavities.[54,55,56,57,58,59,60,61,62,63] Estrogen is a hormone that is present in both men and women, but in significantly higher levels in women. It is responsible for the development and maintenance of female reproductive organs and fertility, as well as other important functions.

The following findings were made from the research conducted on estrogen and cavities, mostly of animal studies:

· As estrogen levels increase, number of cavities increase.

· As estrogen frequency increases, number of cavities increase.

· Different sources of estrogens are additive and possibly synergistic, meaning as more estrogens of different types are given, the effect is even greater than just one type of estrogen, and cavities increase even more.[64]

· The size and overall weight of the submandibular salivary gland is decreased in proportion to the amount of estrogen given – the submandibular gland is a major salivary gland in the mouth, responsible for producing saliva.

## How Does Estrogen Increase Cavities?

Modern research has found that there are estrogen target cells and receptors located within the salivary glands as well as in the gingival tissues (gums).[65] This means that changes in estrogen levels will result in altered function of the salivary glands and other tissues within the mouth. Composition, flow rate and amount of saliva have been shown to fluctuate with changing estrogen levels.[66] In addition, estrogen increases cortisol, and cortisol has been linked with increased cavities.[67]

## Odontoblasts & Estrogen?

In the 1990s, several experiments were conducted in Finland to determine the effect of decreasing estrogen levels on the rate of cavities in rats. This was done by removing the ovaries in both young and mature female rats. It was found that there was an increase in dentin formation in both young and mature rats.[68,69] It is unknown whether the increased dentin formation was a natural result of low estrogen levels or whether it was a secondary response to protect the tooth from injury. Although it is not clear, there is the possibility that odontoblastic function may be affected by estrogen levels. (Remember odonto-blasts make dentin during tooth development and later on to protect a tooth from injury and cavities.)

## Birth Control & Cavities?

In 1979, *Community Dentistry and Oral Epidemiology* published a paper detailing two studies looking at the effects of oral con-traception on cavities.[70]

DMFT = Decayed, Missing, Filled Teeth

DMFS = Decayed, Missing, Filled Surfaces

The study consisted of 6 different groups of women of vary-ing ages taking varying types of birth control pills. The re-searchers did not come to a definitive conclusion, but the fol-lowing was found:

· Of the three older groups of women (the ages were not dis-closed in the study), "all DMFT scores of the 'pill' users were significantly greater than those of the controls…"[71]

· The group of women taking birth control for the longest du-ration (average 3.36 years) had significantly higher DMFT and DMFS numbers than the controls.

## Perimenopause

Estrogen is the dominant hormone in a woman's body for the first two weeks of her menstrual cycle, until ovulation occurs, and then progesterone levels increase for the remaining two weeks. Menopause is associated with a significant decrease in estrogen, however leading up to menopause many women experience elevated levels. In women who do not ovulate, as often occurs for a period of time, and even many years prior to menopause, progesterone levels do not rise as normal and estrogen levels remain elevated as the dominant hormone, potentially resulting in symptoms in the whole body,[72] as well as an increased risk of cavities.

## What About Men and Young Women?

Animal studies show that females, males and young females all experienced increased cavities when exposed to high levels of estrogen. It is inconclusive whether androgens – male hormones such as testosterone – cause an increase in cavities, as there are studies that show no increases and studies that do show increases.[73,74]

## Estrogen Metabolism

Estrogen is metabolized in one of two ways in the body, either pathway 1 or pathway 2.

**Pathway 1:** Estrogen (estradiol) is converted to 2-hydroxyestrone. 2-hydroxyestrone is a very weak estrogen and has little estrogenic activity. This is the ideal pathway of metabolism.

**Pathway 2:** Estrogen (estradiol) is converted to 16 alpha-hydroxyestrone. 16 alpha-hydroxyestrone is a very strong estrogen and has potent estrogenic activity. If estrogen is metabolized by this pathway, the estrogenic activity in the body is increased as opposed to decreased, and this is not ideal.[75]

Essentially an estrogen or estrogen-like substance is broken down to produce either a molecule that is a weaker (pathway 1) or stronger (pathway 2) estrogen. A weaker estrogen will not be as capable of causing an effect on estrogen receptors in the mouth or in rest of the body; a stronger estrogen will be more capable. In an effort to achieve optimal estrogen levels, pathway 1 metabolism is desirable.

## Pathway 1 Inducers and/or Factors Which Decrease Estrogenicity:

· **Indol-3-Carbinol.**[76] This is a substance that is produced by the breakdown of glucosinolate glucobrassicin, which is plentiful in cruciferous vegetables, such as broccoli, cauliflower, Brussels sprouts, kale and collard greens. Indol-3-carbinol is also available as a supplement.[77]

· **Exercise**[78]

## Pathway 2 Inducers and/or Substances that Increase Estrogenicity:[79]

· **Xenoestrogens**. Xenoestrogens are chemicals or natural substances that mimic estrogen, such as bisphenol A[80] and phthalates.[81]

· **Pesticides**

· **Alcohol**

· **Constipation**. Estrogen is eliminated through the feces, and reduced or slow bowel movements can result in the reabsorption of estrogens that should have been removed in the feces.

· **High Ratio of Omega 6 to Omega 3 Fatty Acids**[82]

# Did you Know?

Maca root has traditionally been used for centuries in South America, and is thought to be a potent food to balance hormones. Apparently, maca was so revered that it was used as currency at some points of history. Studies have shown that among other benefits, it can balance the thyroid and sex hormones, namely to increase thyroid hormones and decrease estrogen. Maca root is available as a food, usually dried and powdered, or supplements.[83]

## Beyond Cavities

Elevated estrogen levels are associated with breast cancer. [84,85] Achieving optimal levels of estrogen is not only in the interest of cavity prevention, but for one's overall health, as well.

## Conclusion

The connection that thyroid and estrogen hormones have with cavities makes it clear that tooth environmental factors and internal susceptibility factors are not separate. Thyroid and estrogen hormones affect the target cells involved with the production of saliva, which is a significant tooth environment factor. Any alterations or issues with the hormones will have a cascading effect, leading to alterations or issues related to saliva and potentially increased risk of cavities. Perhaps the future holds further research to explain more of or even a greater connection that thyroid and estrogen hormones have with cavities.

# 9

# A Strong or Susceptible Tooth: Dentin Fluid Flow

"Claude Bernard once stated, "The organism is an entity, a whole from which no single part can be isolated." Can teeth logically be considered apart from the whole body?"

*– Dentinal Fluid Transport[1]*

Within the very inside of a tooth is the pulp. The pulp contains nerves, arteries, veins, lymph, connective tissue cells, collagen, macrophages (immune system component), fibroblasts and odontoblasts (cells that make dentin).[2] One of the functions of the pulp is to provide nutrition and moisture or fluid for the dentin.[3] Remember that dentin is composed of many tiny tubes, and that odontoblasts sit in the pulp with their long arms (Tomes fibers) extending into the dentin tubes. Fluid is circulated by the blood into the pulp of the tooth, and is moved by the odontoblasts from the pulp into the dentin.[4] This moisture or fluid movement from the pulp into the dentin is referred to as the following, all of which mean the same:

- Dentin fluid
- Dentinal fluid
- Dentin fluid flow
- Dentinal fluid flow

Think of this process as a factory assembly line. The blood carries the fluid with nutrients to the pulp. The pulp passes the fluid along to the odontoblasts and the odontoblasts pass it along to the dentin.

**Blood → Pulp → Odontoblast → Dentin**

Picture the following scenario:

A Jacuzzi bathtub is full of water and bubbling away at maximum speed. The water splashes around, and a bit flows out of the bathtub because it is so full and strong. A child comes along and drops an opened disposable ketchup packet into the bathtub. The packet floats around on the surface of the bath, hopping from side to side like someone crowd surfing at a concert. Tiny drops of ketchup leak out of the packet, but are splashed right out of the bathtub, carried by the bubbling water. Ten minutes later, the child's mother comes into the bathroom for her bath and sees the ketchup packet floating on top of the water. She laughs, picks it up and throws it out. She doesn't even notice that it was open, and no obvious signs of ketchup appear in the water.

Now picture a different scenario. The full bathtub that's bubbling away at maximum speed is switched off and the drain plug is pulled. A child comes along and drops an opened disposable ketchup packet into the draining bathtub. There are no bubbles to carry out the tiny droplets of ketchup, and the drops instead fall to the bottom of the tub. Ten minutes later, the child's mother comes into the bathroom and gasps in shock. All the water has drained out of the tub, and the ketchup packet is sitting at the bottom, surrounded by a red line smeared all the way across the tub to the drain. The mother angrily spends the next ten minutes cleaning out the tub.

A tooth that has lots of fluid flow within its dentin is like the full Jacuzzi on high power. Just like the bubbling water kept the ketchup packet from reaching the bottom of the tub, even in the presence of bacterial acids and other potentially damaging factors, abundant dentin fluid flow prevents the cavity-causing acid from entering into the tooth and no cavity occurs. A tooth with lots of fluid flow within the dentin is resistant to cavities[5,6,7,8,9,10,11] and other problems like deep staining, cracking and sensitivity.

A tooth that has little or no fluid flow within its dentin is like the Jacuzzi bathtub that has been turned off and the drain plug pulled. Just like there is no bubbling water to resist the ketchup so it easily reaches the bottom of the tub, there is no fluid flow to resist bacterial acids from entering into the tooth. When bacterial acids enter a tooth, demineralization occurs and a cavity begins or continues progression.

Another way I like to think about dentin fluid flow is to imagine that the tooth is sweating when the fluid flow is abundant. Imagine trying to rub lotion on your body when you are sweating profusely. Not much lotion gets into your skin, right? How about when your skin is dry and cracked? The lotion soaks in right away. The tooth that has little or no fluid flow within its dentin is like dry and cracked skin. Bacterial acids soak right in.

In order to have a strong tooth that is

resistant to bacterial acids there needs to be

abundant dentin fluid flow.

# Dentin Fluid 101

## Dentin fluid serves three purposes:[12]

1. It supplies nutrients for the metabolic functions occurring within teeth, such as the formation of reparative dentin.[13]

2. It functions as a defence mechanism to protect against bacterial acids, as well as sensitivity.[14]

3. It is alkaline, with a pH similar to blood (7.4), and acts as a buffer against acids.[15]

## Speed of Flow

Dentin fluid moves at different speeds. This speed has been measured experimentally using tubes connected to a hydraulic circuit with an adjustable pressure reservoir and measuring device.[16]

## Where is Dental Fluid Found

Dentin fluid flow extends from the pulp to the dentinoenamel junction (DEJ), which is where enamel contacts dentin.

# Parotid Hormone

## Discovery of the Parotid Hormone

It was known back in the early 1900s that substances injected into animals could be found a short while later within the teeth.[17,18] Since those early experiments, numerous studies were conducted and published in dental journals in the United States and Europe detailing experiments to explain the phenomena of dentin fluid flow. Dogs, monkeys and other animals were injected with a variety of substances, such as dyes, antibiotics, glucose and radioactive substances. The substances were injected in a variety of places, including the stomach and skin. Their teeth were sectioned, and varying levels of the injected substances were measured in their teeth. Dyes, antibiotics, glucose and radioactive fluids were all found within the dentin of teeth starting ten to fifteen minutes after injection.[19,20,21,22,23,24,25,26,27]

(I would just like to say that out of respect for the many animals that sacrificed their lives for dental research, let's show our gratitude and love by learning from the research so that their lives were not lost in vain.)

This dye penetration is not something that can be seen externally – it is not like staining of the enamel, for example. After the dyes were injected into various body parts, the teeth were extracted and drilled open. Inside the teeth, the dye was visible, but not externally. A substance was isolated that could stimulate more injected dye to be found in the dentin of teeth.

**Dye injected into body + No Substance**

**= No Dye found in Teeth**

**Dye injected into body + Special Substance**

**= Dye Absorbed in Teeth**

This special substance is found in the parotid gland, which is a major salivary gland in the mouth that secretes saliva. The substance was named the parotid hormone. When lots of parotid hormone is given, lots of dye penetrates into the dentin of teeth; when the parotid gland is removed from animals, no dye penetrates into the teeth.

**Special Substance = Parotid Hormone**[28]

# Parotid Hormone & Cavities

Weeks before cavities are detected in teeth, the first change noted is reduced fluid flow into the dentin. Animals with low levels of parotid hormone production and therefore low levels of dentin fluid flow, experience a higher rate of cavities. High levels of parotid hormone production and high levels of dentin fluid flow result in a significantly lower rate of cavities.[29]

↑ **Parotid Hormone**

= ↑ **Dentin Fluid Flow**

= **Tooth is Protected From Cavities**

↓ **Parotid Hormone**

= ↓ **Dentin Fluid Flow**

= **Tooth is Susceptible to Cavities**

(Remember to think of dentin fluid flow as the tooth sweating and no bacterial acids can enter, like no lotion gets absorbed in sweating skin.)

## Dentin Fluid & Staining

Experiments were conducted on teeth with very little dentin fluid flow. Dyes applied to the enamel on the outside part of the tooth were able to deeply penetrate into the enamel of the teeth. Teeth that had high levels of dentin fluid flow also had dyes applied to the enamel. These teeth showed little or no dye penetration into the enamel. (This is now *external* dye penetration – the esthetic type.)

↑ **Dentin Fluid = ↓ External Staining**

↓ **Dentin Fluid = ↑ External Staining**

## Parotid Hormone Regulation

The parotid hormone is regulated by the hypothalamus. The hypothalamus is the "master gland" located in the brain. The hypothalamus can either up-regulate or down-regulate the parotid hormone. The hypothalamus sends signals that can result in lots of parotid hormone production (up-regulation) or limited amounts of parotid hormone production (down-regulation).[30,31,32] Researchers found that parotid hormone levels increased when animals were given hypothalamus-thalamus tissue extracts.

**Hypothalamus Signals for Up-Regulation of the Parotid Gland = ↑ Parotid Hormone = ↑ Dentin Fluid = Tooth is Protected From Cavities**

**Hypothalamus Signals for Down-Regulation of the Parotid Gland = ↓ Parotid Hormone = ↓ Dentin Fluid = Tooth is Susceptible to Cavities**

# Did You Know?

The most recent significant scientific breakthrough for the systemic prevention of cavities occurred in 2005, with the cloning of the DNA that codes for the amino acid sequence of the parotid hormone.[33] The cloning of animal DNA to produce parotid hormone opens up a possibility to create a new approach to the prevention of cavities. Like a diabetic who is given the hormone insulin, there are rumors that the future of cavity prevention is giving people parotid hormone. Although that sounds exciting, it may continue to remain just a rumor, like the rumor of a vaccine against MS bacteria to prevent cavities. In this book, I will tell you how to naturally increase your parotid hormone without waiting for external supplementation to be developed!

## Fluoride & Dentin Fluid Flow

In addition to the topical abilities of fluoride to harden teeth and cavities,[34] fluoride has been shown experimentally to stimulate an increase of dentin fluid.[35]

## Parotid Hormone 101

· The speed at which dyes or other injectables show up in the dentin of teeth varies significantly. Some substances show up more quickly while other substances take longer.

· The amount of penetration into teeth varies significantly. Some substances have a greater penetration into the dentin of teeth than others. In other words, some substances can stimulate parotid hormone production and help a tooth resist cavities, while other substances do not stimulate parotid hormone production and do not possess the ability to help a tooth resist cavities.

- The amount of penetration into the dentin of teeth is not dependent on the pH or acid level of the substance or the pH of the mouth.

- Two minutes after eating, parotid hormone is detectable, peaking at ten to twenty minutes after eating, and slowly decreases over the two hours following a meal.[36]

## Parotid Hormone as Protection

Parotid hormone production and dentin fluid flow appear to be a form of protection for teeth. Mealtime and immediately following are when the teeth are most exposed to potentially damaging conditions caused by bacterial acids, as they feed on sugars. Parotid hormone peaks at this time to resist the influx of acid that could lead to a cavity.

To Recap:

- A susceptible tooth is one that has low levels of dentin fluid flow.

- A strong and resistant tooth is one that has high levels of dentin fluid flow.

Susceptible to what? Cavities, of course, which is what this book is focused on. However, a susceptible tooth is also prone to breakage, cracking, staining and sensitivity.

The goal is to have a high level of dentin fluid flow. How to do so is covered in the following two chapters:

Autonomic Nervous System

Food

(If you would like to learn more about dentin fluid flow, I highly recommend reading the book, *Dentinal Fluid Transport*, by Ralph Steinman and John Leonora and condensed by Clyde Roggenkamp. This book contains one hundred research articles that show the discovery of the parotid hormone and how it affects teeth, as well as the research behind the systemic connection with cavities.)

# 10

## A Strong or Susceptible Tooth: Autonomic Nervous System

I magine... You hear from a friend that a position at their company has just become available. It's your dream job! You apply and get an interview. Every day for the two weeks before your interview, you practice in the mirror what you are going to say, and you are sure you will do really well.

You sit in front of the three people interviewing you. All six eyes across the desk are staring at you, waiting for your answer to their question.

You don't hear their question. You ask them to repeat the question. You hear it and begin answering, but lose focus part way through your answer and stop talking. The interviewers make a note on their papers, "Can't focus." What is happening inside your body? The hypothalamus in your brain has stimulated the parotid gland in your mouth to produce parotid hormone.[1,2] The odontoblasts inside your teeth start pumping fluid from the pulp into your dentin, and no bacterial acids enter your tooth. Your tooth is protected from cavities![3,4,5,6] Yay! You are dismissed from the job interview and told that they are looking for someone with more ability to focus. (That was a sarcastic "yay" in case you wondered.)

And you wake up from your nightmare! You go off to the interview for real and as the three interviewers' eyes are on you, you answer their questions with professionalism, focus and intelligence. You ace the interview and are accepted on the spot for the job. As you shake hands and leave, the interviewers say that they are impressed with how sharp and focused you are. What was happening inside your body? Your hypothalamus in your brain knew you were in an emergency situation and stopped any focus on stimulating your parotid gland.[7,8,9] The teeth can wait! All focus was put on increasing your A game. Your eyes could see clearly, your mind was sharp and your thoughts came quickly. When one of the interviewers dropped their pen, your muscles reacted in perfect coordination and you caught it mid-fall. On the drive home, you took a deep breath and turned your favorite radio station on to celebrate your success. Your hypothalamus knew you were out of the emergency situation and its attention turned to making sure your teeth are in a protected state so you don't get a cavity!

## Autonomic Nervous System 101

The hypothalamus controls the autonomic nervous system, which consists of the sympathetic and parasympathetic nervous systems. The sympathetic nervous system is responsible for our stress response – it is sometimes referred to as the fight or flight response. It gets your heart beating faster, your blood pumping faster and your pupils dilate so you can see better. It prepares you to battle a sabre-toothed tiger, or these days, to say a speech at work. Your digestion slows and all your body's focus is on preparing you for whatever stress (good or bad, physical or emotional[10]) is happening. Digestion, liver filtration and other important but non-emergency-type functions are stopped or slowed and picked up again when the stress is stopped. When the stress is stopped, the parasympathetic nervous system is activated and the important but non-emergency type functions controlled by the parasympathetic nervous system are focused on.[11]

There are three main hormones involved with the stress response. Adrenaline (also called epinephrine), noradrenaline (also called norepinephrine) and cortisol are all produced by the adrenal glands in response to a stressful situation. (Hydrocortisone is synthetic cortisol, often administered as a medication.) Adrenaline and noradrenaline are immediately produced, almost instantaneously, while cortisol takes longer. Adrenaline, and to a large extent noradrenaline, are directly released from the adrenal glands, like a reflex, without thinking. Cortisol, on the other hand, is not a reflex type of release. The brain senses the need for cortisol and then there is a chain reaction of signals sent from the hypothalamus to the pituitary gland to the adrenal glands.[12]

These hormones are lifesaving. If you are driving in a car and a child darts out in front of you, you can slam on the brakes immediately; the fight or flight response plays a major role in such a great ability. Almost instantly your heart beats faster, your eyes open wide and you are very alert; the hormones adrenaline and noradrenaline are to thank.

# Cortisol

Cortisol plays an important role in less instantaneously stressful situations. Like playing a sport or competing in a race, saying a speech or asking your boss for a raise; also emotional circumstances like getting married, getting a divorce, dealing with children, coworkers, etc. Cortisol is released to make sure you are having a peak performance, that you're alert when you're up to bat and not drowsy during an interview. The Parasympathetic Nervous System shuts down excessive cortisol production, though a small amount is constantly produced, which is necessary for healthy functioning.

## Cortisol also has the following effects:

- Immune suppression.[13]
- Bone formation is reduced.
- Calcium absorption is reduced.
- Collagen is removed from tissues and collagen formation is inhibited.[14] (Remember teeth contain collagen.)
- Elevated cortisol levels are associated with decreased fertility, which makes sense because fertility is not a bodily function that is necessary during emergency situations.[15] Additionally, cortisol can enter the placenta and affect the growth of a fetus.[16]

# Interesting Study

Dental students inflicted small wounds on the roof of their mouths at two different times of the year. The first was during their summer break and the second was right before a major exam, a source of significant stress for the dental students. The wounds made before the exam took an average of three days longer to heal, and the students produced 68% less interleukin, a component of the immune system.[17]

# Cavities & the Autonomic Nervous System

It has been known since the mid-1900s that stress hormones increase the rate of cavities.[18,19,20,21,22,23] Today it is understood that the greater susceptibility to cavities is due to decreased dentin fluid flow. Activation of the sympathetic nervous system results in down-regulation of the parotid hormone and reduced dentin fluid flow within teeth.[24] Parasympathetic stimulation results in increased fluid movement into the dentin from the pulp, resulting in significant protection from cavities.

**Parasympathetic Nervous System Activation**

**= Strong Tooth**

**Sympathetic Nervous System Activation**

**= Susceptible Tooth**

Fluid flow within the dentin of teeth is a protective mechanism. The increased levels of parotid hormone within minutes of feeding followed by a gradual decrease over a two-hour period indicates that the body is attempting to protect the teeth during the most potentially harmful time. This is a time when food sources for bacteria are highest, and when the acid production from bacteria is the greatest.

As a form of protection for teeth during and after feeding, it makes perfect sense that parasympathetic nervous system activation increases parotid hormone production, and sympathetic nervous system activation reduces parotid hormone levels. This is because feeding is a time when parasympathetic activation is highest, or at least it should be.

This is a great process for us. It allows us to perform at our peak during a game of tennis. You want your body to focus energy on good eyesight and fast reflexes, and not on digesting food or filtering your blood. In times of stress, protecting teeth from cavities will in no way help with the stressful situation. No one wants their body to be focusing on dentin fluid flow and protecting their teeth while they are saying a speech, asking for a raise or competing in a sporting event. We all want our bodies to focus on peak performance (sympathetic nervous system) and then deal with protecting our teeth later (parasympathetic nervous system).

## Cortisol & Salivary Glands

Cortisol decreases the size of the salivary glands.[25] Remember cortisol diminishes the activity of any unnecessary bodily functions during a stressful situation. This is often accomplished by reducing blood flow to the area and constricting the permeability of an organ or gland. It's as if cortisol ties an elastic band around any part of the body that is not considered important during stress and this starves the area of blood flow. It is believed that cortisol constricts blood flow to the teeth and salivary glands. Maintaining an adequate supply of blood to the pulp is thought to be a main predictor of whether dentin will be able to remineralize or not.[26]

## When It Rains, It Pours

I've lost count of the number of times I've heard the statement, "When it rains, it pours," or some similar remark in my office. Often people say, "This is the last thing I need in my life right now." My heart goes out to these people because I know they are already under a lot of stress. Health issues with themselves or a loved one, marital troubles, a sick or dying parent, behavioral problems with children, just to name a few of the stressful issues experienced in modern society. Excessive sympathetic nervous system activation, combined with increased incidence of clenching and grinding, changes in food habits and immune system depletion can result in some tremendous damage to teeth. I hope that everyone, especially those experiencing chronic stress, can find some peace in their lives.

## How to Know If You Have Elevated Cortisol?

Salivary cortisol levels are measured by a simple swab of saliva. Speak to your healthcare practitioner about testing. You can also purchase some tests online to do yourself.

# How to Achieve Optimal Balance of the Autonomic Nervous System

### 1. Balanced Fatty Acids

Consuming omega-3 fatty acids has been shown to decrease cortisol levels, and high levels of unbalanced omega-6 fatty acids increase cortisol.[27,28] Foods high in omega3 fatty acids include:

Cold water fish, especially salmon, herring, mackerel, sardines

Hemp seeds

Pumpkin seeds

Walnuts

Flax seeds

Chia seeds

## 2. Magnesium

Increased magnesium consumption is associated with decreased cortisol levels.[29,30]

Good Sources of magnesium:[31]

- Green plants and herbs, including kelp, dulse, dandelion, burdock root, chickweed and nettles.

- Nuts such as almonds, cashews, Brazil nuts, pecans, walnuts

- Mineral water

- Sea salt

- Supplements

Vitamins E and B6 are necessary for magnesium absorption.[32]

## 3. Massage Therapy[33]

## 4. Sleep

Sleep deprivation increases cortisol levels.[34]

## 5. Reduce Caffeine

Caffeine increases cortisol levels.[35]

## 6. Have Fun

Laughter and humor decrease cortisol levels.[36]

## 7. Music

Listening to music you enjoy can decrease cortisol levels.[37]

## 8. Exercise

Exercised animals have increased dentin fluid flow and decreased cavities. In 1960, the School of Dentistry at Loma Linda University published a study about two groups of rats that were fed the exact same cavity-inducing diet. One group was in a large cage where there was space for them to move and run around, and the other group was in a cage with wires that restricted them from moving around. The rats that were restricted had 3.25 times more cavities than the rats fed the same diet but that were exercised.[38]

How can this be? Remember, dentin fluid flow is reduced during periods of sympathetic stimulation, and the animals in confinement experienced higher levels of stress.

## 9. Dance

Why not dance more? Movement, music and fun, so much good all combined together. What a thought – that dancing is good for your teeth! In fact, dancing has been shown to decrease cortisol levels![39]

## 10. Decrease Stress

Stress is a rather immeasurable and subjective matter, and decreasing stress is a very personal action plan.

I know a woman who was taking exceptional care of her teeth and eating an incredibly nutritious diet. But she was continually experiencing new, actively progressing cavities. After I explained to her the connection our autonomic nervous system has with our teeth, she decided to use self-hypnosis and visualize her teeth healing. And it worked! There is no way I could have come up with self-hypnosis as a solution for her, but she knew what was best for herself.

I think a good place to start is to acknowledge that you have excessive stress in your life, and make sure you have fun doing something every day.

## Children, Stress & Cavities

Is Your Child Experiencing Stress?

In 2010, there was research published in *Social Science and Medicine*, detailing the findings of two large studies comparing salivary cortisol levels and cavity rates in San Francisco kindergarten-aged children of varying socioeconomic status. Not only did they find that many children had high levels of cortisol, but there was a proportional increase in cavities with increased cortisol levels. The higher the cortisol, the more cavities, enamel softness and cavity-causing bacteria were found.[40]

## Stress as a Piece of the Puzzle

Chronic stress is a common occurrence in modern society. Even with a healthy diet, if someone has excessive sympathetic nervous system activation, their teeth will be susceptible to cavities. So often I hear people say something along the lines of, "I don't understand why I get cavities, I don't eat sugar, and I eat so healthily." Having high levels of stress offers another piece to the puzzle. (And make sure you don't experience even more stress because you don't understand why you are getting cavities.) It is remarkable to think that stress can increase one's cavity risk. The link emotions have with cavities is not a commonly thought about or discussed risk factor. However, I think it really hits home the point that when one naturally prevents and remineralizes cavities, they will experience great improvements in their life. It may not be easy to reduce the stress in your life, but I promise your teeth won't be the only thing thanking you.

# 11

# A Strong or Susceptible Tooth: Food

From a very old dental school textbook about the rapid increase in cavities experienced in society by a shift from traditional to modern foods:

"In the future, oral care, brushing of the teeth, and regular dental treatment will have to take the place of the former caries immunity."

*– Histopathology of the Teeth and their Surrounding Structures, 1939* [1]

As a dentist, I see the general public, and the general public is made up of a mix of people wishing to follow wildly different diet protocols. A dental office is not a place where similarly minded diet followers gather. Similarly minded diet followers gather together in online groups like you'd find on Facebook. A dental office is more like a market square where people of all beliefs gather together, and where people following various diets are welcome to come for assistance to improve their health. For me to promote one and only one type of diet would be less than ideal for a number of reasons. First of all, I know it is possible for numerous diets to provide people with good oral health because I have seen evidence of that with my own two eyes. Secondly, I would be limiting myself to helping a subset of the population and that is not my intention.

Although there is not just one food or one particular diet that will naturally prevent and remineralize cavities, perhaps there is one particular diet that is best for you, and I highly recommend you follow that diet. If you have cavities or dental problems, I encourage you to entertain the idea that the diet you are following could benefit from some changes ranging from small tweaks to a complete overhaul.

I also highly recommend seeking the advice of a nutritionist, dietician, other professional, and/or doing your own research to find the foods and diet that best suits your needs and desires. This book is not intended to provide readers with a comprehensive list of foods to consume. Rather my goal is to educate the reader to understand why and how foods affect teeth and cavities. Like teaching someone how to fish as opposed to simply giving fish, I want the reader to be able to continually make the best choices for themselves and their family, no matter what foods and diets are popular at the time.

Recap:

Suppressed dentin fluid flow = susceptible tooth = greater incidence of cavities

Abundant dentin fluid flow = strong/unsusceptible tooth = reduced incidence of cavities

Many different substances have been tested for their effects on dentin fluid flow and cavity incidence. The notable substances I will elaborate on are:

Sucrose

Minerals (Zinc, Molybdenum, Chromium)

Carbamoyl Phosphate

## Sucrose

Studies show that sucrose consistently has the **greatest ability to decrease dentin fluid flow and increase incidence of**

**cavities.**[2] Consuming sucrose results in a tooth that is susceptible to cavities.

What is sucrose?

Sucrose is a disaccharide.

Di = two

Saccharide = sugar.

Sucrose is a molecule made up of two separate sugars, a glucose and a fructose. Sucrose is what we know as table sugar or just normal sugar, and any variation of sugar, like icing sugar, confectioners' sugar, etc. Sugar is also informally used to refer to anything sweet, even though it might not actually be sucrose. For example, one might say that pop has a lot of sugar in it, while technically it might have corn syrup in it, or people talk about having high blood sugar levels, which is what a diabetic measures, while technically they are talking about the level of glucose in the blood. In our bodies, sucrose is broken down into its constituent parts, a glucose and a fructose molecule. The glucose is then transported in the blood (and will contribute to high blood "sugar") and will be used as either an energy source or stored as fat. The fructose must first be broken down by the liver before it is used as an energy source or stored as fat.

## Blood-Glucose & Tooth Susceptibility

Sucrose suppresses dentin fluid and increases susceptibility to cavities; high blood-glucose levels do this, as well. This means that anything that increases blood-glucose or "blood sugar" will decrease dentin fluid and leave teeth susceptible to cavities.

It makes sense that high blood-glucose levels suppress dentin fluid movement because part of the function of the sympathetic nervous system is to increase blood-glucose so that it can be used by the body for energy. Remember the sympathetic nervous system is responsible for actions relating to emergency and high-energy needs. For instance, when you are playing a game of tennis, you need higher glucose levels in your blood for energy to play a good game. Emergency and high-energy times are not when the body should be focusing on preventing cavities, thus the high blood-glucose signals that the parotid hormone should not waste energy on cavity prevention. However, excessive blood-glucose levels during non-emergency times means dentin fluid flow is suppressed when the teeth really should be in a protective state. In other words, if you have high blood-glucose levels while sitting on a couch, your dentin behaves the same way as if you are running a marathon. Chronic elevation of blood-glucose is a common issue in modern society, and will result in suppressed dentin fluid, allowing for teeth to accept the acid produced by bacteria. Chronic elevation of blood glucose is associated with Type 2 diabetes and cardiovascular disease,[3] both of which are increasing in prevalence.

# High Blood Sugar

## = Suppressed Dentin Fluid

## = Increased Susceptibility to Cavities

The glycemic index is a measure of how a substance affects blood sugar/glucose levels. The number goes from 1 to 100 where 100 is pure glucose. Foods like bread, potatoes, fruit and rice can also increase blood-glucose, although obviously not as much as pure sugar. Any diabetic or pre-diabetic will likely have higher blood-sugar levels after consuming the same foods as a non-diabetic. To prevent spiking your blood-glucose levels, it is best to eat foods low on the glycemic index, and combine foods high on the glycemic index with fat or protein. Fat and protein slows the speed of absorption of the sugar into the blood and prevents a sudden increase in blood-glucose. We almost instinctively know to combine high-glycemic foods with foods that will help prevent a spike in blood sugar, for example, eating bread with butter or a baked potato with sour cream and bacon.

The following are all sweeteners capable of increasing blood-sugar:

Cane juice, dehydrated cane juice, cane juice solids, cane juice crystals, dextrin, maltodextrin, dextran, barley malt, beet sugar, corn syrup, corn syrup solids, caramel, buttered syrup, carob syrup, brown sugar, date sugar, malt syrup, diatase, diatastic malt, fruit juice, fruit juice concentrate, dehydrated fruit juice, fruit juice crystals, golden syrup, turbinado, sorghum syrup, refiner's syrup, ethyl maltol, yellow sugar.[4]

## High-Fructose Corn Syrup

High-fructose corn syrup has been implicated as a major source of cavities.[5] High-fructose corn syrup is found in many products, and is often labelled as glucose-fructose.

# Whole Food Sweeteners

Whole food natural sweeteners can also increase blood-glucose levels and negatively affect fluid flow within teeth, but unlike refined sugars, they at least provide some nutritional benefits while doing so. Natural sweeteners should be consumed in moderation.

Examples of whole food sweeteners include:[6]

### 1. Raw Honey

Raw honey is known to have antibiotic, antibacterial and antimicrobial properties, and also contains antioxidants, vitamins, minerals and enzymes.

### 2. Molasses

Blackstrap molasses is a good source of iron and calcium.

### 3. Artichoke Syrup

Artichoke syrup has a low-glycemic index and is high in inulin, which feeds good gut bacteria.

### 4. Lucuma Powder

Lucuma is an excellent source of beta carotene, vitamins B1 and B2 and has a low-glycemic index.

### 5. Stevia

Stevia has no calories and no glycemic impact. It is usually found as a granular powder that looks like sugar but tastes much sweeter. You can also grow it as a plant and use the plant leaves to sweeten foods.

## Sugar at Mealtime

Modern dentistry has long promoted eating sugary foods with meals as opposed to snacking on them throughout the day as an important strategy to protect against cavities by preventing a drop in pH (increased acidity). This advice also holds true for protecting the internal state of the tooth and ensuring higher levels of dentin fluid.[7] Even better, instead of consuming foods that are bad for your teeth (and body) at meals, reducing these foods in general will be the most protective to your teeth (and body).

Sugar is linked with cavities, from both a tooth-environment and tooth-susceptibility perspective. Sugar creates a harsh mouth environment, providing food for the cavity-causing bacteria, which in turn produce acid and dissolve the minerals out of the tooth.[8] From the tooth-susceptibility perspective, sugar reduces dentin fluid flow resulting in enamel and dentin that readily soaks in the bacterial acids. Clearly, sugar consumption increases one's susceptibility to cavities on many levels.

# Minerals

In the numerous experiments done on dentin fluid flow, the minerals that were studied consistently resulted in an **increase in dentin fluid** flow and a reduction in cavities. When added to other substances that could stimulate dentin fluid flow, the minerals potentiated the effects and offered even greater protection to cavities.

The minerals studied were chromium, zinc and molybdenum, which are also termed trace elements.

# Molybdenum

The main function of molybdenum is to help breakdown amino acids.

**Sources:**[9]

- Organ meats
- Leafy green vegetables
- Whole grains
- Beans

# Zinc

Zinc is important in immune function, collagen production and wound healing. It plays a role in carbohydrate and protein metabolism, normal fetal development, and protects against vision loss.[10] Zinc is also involved with the normal production and action of insulin. A deficiency impairs blood-glucose regulation, resulting in additional susceptibility to cavities.[11]

**Signs of zinc deficiency:**[12]

- Hair loss
- Weight loss
- Delayed wound healing
- Chronic infection
- Rough skin
- Skin rashes
- Poor appetite
- Depression
- Mental lethargy

**Sources:**[13]

- Fish
- Oysters
- Beans
- Whole grains
- Meats
- Pumpkin seeds
- Nuts
- Eggs

# Chromium

Chromium is essential for proper maintenance of blood-glucose levels. A deficiency, even of a mild degree, impairs the effectiveness of insulin, resulting in elevated blood-glucose levels. Chromium deficiency is associated with Type 2 Diabetes, Metabolic Syndrome, and blood sugar regulation problems. It is estimated that between 25-50% of the population in the United States is deficient in chromium. Antacids, corticosteroids, Proton-pump inhibitors and H2 blockers decrease the absorption of chromium from the gut. Refined sugar is said to deplete the body of chromium because it requires chromium to be metabolized, but does not provide any chromium to replace it.[14]

**Signs of deficiency:**[15]

- Anxiety
- Fatigue
- Delayed wound healing
- Decreased growth in children

**Sources:**[16]

- Nutritional yeast
- Brewer's yeast
- Molasses
- Black pepper
- Meat
- Organ meat
- Whole grains
- Broccoli
- Grapes

- Raw onions
- Romaine lettuce
- Tomatoes

## Other Minerals

Although molybdenum, zinc and chromium are the three specific minerals studied in reference to dentin fluid flow, other minerals must also be considered as well. There is extensive interaction with one another, and deficiency or excess of one can negatively affect others. Some nutrients are necessary for others to be properly absorbed, assimilated or metabolized. Thus, although research is only available for how zinc, chromium and molybdenum affect teeth, it is necessary to have optimal levels of numerous minerals in order to ensure abundant dentin fluid and protection from cavities.

**Mineral deficiency**

**= Decreased dentin fluid**

**= Increased cavities**

Minerals can be depleted or malabsorbed through certain systemic conditions, diets and even emotions. Alcohol, stress, excessive exercise, menstruation, poor digestion and illnesses can all affect mineral levels in the body.[17]

# Carbamoyl Phosphate

In the studies of dentin fluid flow, carbamoyl phosphate consistently showed the **greatest increase in dentin fluid** flow, compared to all other studied substances. Either alone or with added components like eggshells, carbamoyl phosphate was most able to prevent cavities due to significant induction of dentin fluid flow within teeth.

**Carbamoyl Phosphate + EggShell Meal + Minerals**
**(Zinc, Molybdenum, Chromium)**
**= Greatest Fluid Flow**

Carbamoyl phosphate is not a food, nor is it consumed in foods or taken in supplements. Carbamoyl phosphate is an essential component in the production of energy within the body. Remember that within the body, energy (ATP) production occurs within the mitochondria of a cell and involves the production of a free radical used in the signaling process for physiological functions including MMP activation. Carbamoyl phosphate is not only a critical step in this process, but it can also behave as a mitochondrial antioxidant since it contains extra electrons to donate to the natural free radicals produced during energy production. Thus, carbamoyl phosphate can reduce levels of natural free radicals.[18]

Although laboratory-fabricated antioxidants which have been targeted specifically to affect the mitochondria, are most able to decrease free radicals within the mitochondria, normal, naturally occurring antioxidants have also been shown to decrease mitochondrial free radicals.[19]

# Antioxidant Sources[20]

### Glutathione

- Fruits
- Vegetables
- Freshly cooked meat
- Lipoic acid increases levels of glutathione
- N-acetyl-L-cysteine (NAC) increases glutathione

### Vitamin E

- Raw vegetable oils
- Nuts
- Nut butters
- Rice bran oil
- Barley
- Leafy green vegetables

### Vitamin C

- Fruits, especially citrus and cranberries
- Vegetables, especially red peppers, broccoli, cabbage, tomatoes
- Camu camu berries
- Flavonoids increase effectiveness of vitamin C

### Coenzyme Q10

- Seafood
- Organ meats

# Nutrition & Developing Teeth

In 1995, a paper published in the *Journal of American Clinical Nutrition* detailed two studies involving 285 children aged three to nine, and 209 children aged six to eleven months who were followed over a four-year period of time. The children were from poor suburbs of Peru and were categorized as being either chronically malnourished, having one acute episode of malnutrition, or well nourished.

The researchers studied the DEFT number of each child. (DEFT is Decayed, Extracted, Filled Teeth.) The children were all fed a diet that regained their health from either being chronically or one-time acutely malnourished.

The researchers found that the malnourished children had delayed eruption and exfoliation (falling out) of their deciduous teeth, meaning their baby teeth did not come in or fall out in a timely manner.

The study also showed that the children who had been chronically malnourished had a significantly higher number of decayed, extracted or filled teeth (DEFT), followed by the one-time malnourished children, with the well-nourished children having the lowest number of DEFT.

The young children aged six to eleven months who were followed for four or more years, showed a similar pattern to those who had been chronically malnourished, and had the highest number of decayed, extracted or filled teeth (DEFT) in both their deciduous *and permanent teeth*, followed by the children with just one acute episode of malnutrition and the well-nourished children experienced the least number. Even though the teeth were not in the mouth during the time of malnutrition, they were still negatively affected years later. [21]

Not only does diet affect cavities, but diet affects FUTURE cavities. Diet and nutrition at an early age influences one's susceptibility to cavities at a later date. Remarkably, these studies showed that even *one* episode of nutritional deprivation at an early age can increase one's susceptibility to cavities in the future.

## Nutritional Deprivation is Not Just About Calories

Nutritional deprivation does not only include calorie restriction, but also includes having a diet that provides sufficient (or excessive) calories but not enough vitamins and minerals.

"When a person is not getting enough food or not getting the right sort of food, malnutrition is just around the corner. Even if people get enough to eat, they will become malnourished if the food they eat does not provide the proper amounts of micronutrients – vitamins and minerals – to meet daily nutritional requirements." –World Food Programme[22]

# Why Do Children Get More Cavities Than Adults?

The developing tooth is much more susceptible to cavities than an already-formed tooth.[23] During tooth development, the metabolic demands on the tooth are the greatest they will ever be, and this increased activity within the tooth puts it at higher risk of developing cavities.[24] Imagine that you have a to-do list of three things that you need to accomplish in one day. Then imagine that you have a to-do list of one hundred things that you need to accomplish in one day. Which day are you more at risk of making a mistake in your tasks? Of course, the day that you have many more tasks to do is the day when you are more likely to make a mistake. This is like a developing tooth that has so many activities occurring within it – the many different parts of the tooth are forming, all while still working to protect the tooth from harm and cavities. There is so much going on at this time in a tooth's life that it is most likely to make a mistake that can result in a cavity. Even though the same conditions that caused a cavity in a child may still exist in the adult, the adult may not necessarily develop a cavity.

Not only are developing teeth more susceptible to cavities, but cavities in developing teeth progress more rapidly.[25] Studies have shown that cavities in developing teeth progress up to *ten* times faster than cavities in already formed teeth.[26] This is an important consideration when attempting to remineralize cavities in children.

With age, more and more dentin is produced (secondary or reparative dentin) for a variety of reasons, such as to repair damage or for protection from external stimuli.[27,28,29] This increased amount of dentin can take up space within the pulp, which is why older adults often have much smaller pulp chambers and canals than younger individuals. The increased production of dentin over time also results in more stiff and dense dentin.[30] The increased density and stiffness of dentin in older teeth results in greater protection from cavities, but increased risk of fracture because the teeth are more brittle.[31] Additionally, there is evidence that the collagen within teeth develops more cross-linkages, making the teeth stronger, less susceptible to decay, but more brittle.[32] Think of an old pair of jeans that keeps on getting patched up. With so many patches, the jeans aren't as likely to tear anymore, although they also feel a little stiffer to wear.

## Dentin Formation

The metabolic activities occurring within developing teeth involve the transfer of proteins and minerals between odontoblasts and dentin. Dentin fluid flow plays a significant role in this process, and reduced dentin fluid during tooth development will result in the abnormal formation of dentin. This abnormal formation is not something that is visible to the eye or

X-ray, but can result in increased susceptibility to cavities for the duration of the life of the affected tooth.[33] Reduced dentin fluid flow has been shown to negatively affect the formation of both primary and secondary dentin (dentin that is made during tooth development as well as dentin made afterwards).[34,35] Decreased fluid flow even *prior to eruption* of teeth is associated with increased cavities.[36] Studies have shown that diets high in sucrose (which decreases dentin fluid flow) during tooth development will negatively affect the formation of dentin, and the teeth will be permanently more susceptible to cavities.[37,38] When sucrose, corn syrup, dextromaltose and fructose are given to animals PRIOR to the teeth being present in the mouth, upon eruption the teeth are twice as likely to get cavities compared to animals given only water or lactose.[39] Once a tooth appears in the mouth, it continues primary dentin development for 3 years (for permanent teeth.)[40]

Reduced dentin fluid in a child has some pretty hefty repercussions. Not only will their teeth be immediately susceptible to decay, but their teeth will have impaired development and structuring of dentin that puts them at higher risk of decay in the future.

The idea that one's susceptibility to cavities can be related to food that they ate as a baby and young child is a perfect example of how complex the etiology of cavities is. It is simply not possible to look at what your neighbor is doing who has healthy teeth and assume that if you do the same thing and eat and drink the same foods, you too will have healthy teeth. Often I see parents who are shocked that their child has cavities when neither parent has ever had a problem with cavities; husbands and wives who eat the same diet and one continually struggles with decay, while the other effortlessly has healthy teeth.

If you have the opportunity to affect a child's development of teeth, I highly recommend helping set that child up for successful prevention and remineralization of cavities in the present and future by ensuring they have abundant fluid flow within their teeth. I say that it is giving the child one of the greatest gifts – the gift of strong, healthy teeth that will help resist decay for their lifetime.

If, however, that "ship has sailed," and the child or adult has teeth that are susceptible to cavities, I encourage you not to dwell on the past. Having regrets for what you could have done or resenting someone for what you think they should have done will not get you any closer to having the healthy mouth you desire for yourself and your family. You don't have to throw in the towel if you or a loved one has a higher susceptibility to cavities due to impaired tooth development (or any other reason). So often people say they have soft teeth and take it to mean they have a life sentence of cavities. Remember that the cause of cavities is multifactorial, and tooth structure resulting from early nutrition, dentin fluid or even genetics is only a part of the whole picture. There are many other factors besides tooth structure developed from early years that determines whether a cavity will develop. If you feel as though you or your child has an increased susceptibility to cavities, there are so many things you can do to prevent and remineralize cavities. It will quite possibly be more challenging for you than for someone who has had different development of their teeth, but it is possible, and certainly well worth the effort.

## Resurgence of Old Prevention Strategies

From *Sturdevant's Art & Science of Operative Dentistry*:
"The mechanism of caries reduction is not entirely understood and apparently not fully explained by either the use of fluoride or a reduction in sucrose consumption. Thus, other factors once considered to be of little importance, in fact, may have a considerable impact on caries."[41]

Some fascinating studies were published prior to the Second World War relating to food and cavities. The following details two such publications: [42]

In 1928, the *Journal of the American Medical Association* published a paper from the Department of Pediatrics and Dentistry at the State University of Iowa.

It described an unplanned and unusual set of findings involving twenty-eight diabetic children having been seen regularly in the medical clinic and dental department for six months. It was found that these children had quite extensive areas of arrested decay in their teeth, while most of them had initially been found with large, actively progressing cavities.

The only changes these children had experienced were the introduction of insulin for their diabetes and a change in diet.

The children were fed a diet extremely low in sugar and consisted of a daily quart of milk and cream, butter, eggs, meat, cod liver oil, vegetables and fruit.

The following year, in 1929, the *Journal of the American Medical Association* again published a paper from the Department of Pediatrics and Dentistry at the State University of Iowa, this time detailing several experimental studies involving non-diabetic children.

The first study involved children with extensive cavities, "the activity being obviously demonstrable by the softness of the exposed dentine."[43] These children, who were being treated in the orthopedic ward, were fed a diet similar to the diabetic children, but, of course, received no insulin: a quart of milk and cream, butter, eggs, meat, cod liver oil, vegetables and fruit daily. In two months the cavities were remineralized, "the arrest being evidenced by the change in the consistency of the dentine from the initial state to one of stony hardness, with no advance in the destructive process."[44]

The children who continued to attend the clinic but no longer had their diets controlled were found to have new, active cavities several months later.

The researchers then studied children with active cavities in their home environment. The mothers were instructed to ensure the children had daily one quart of whole milk, one egg, a teaspoon of cod liver oil, one ounce of butter, one orange or tomato juice and two or more servings of succulent vegetables and fruit. They could eat whatever else they wanted, as long as they ate the prescribed foods. Some of the mothers said that indeed their children ate candy and other sugary foods. Some of the children ate a diet high in fat and low in carbohydrates and others had a diet high in carbohydrates and protein and low in fat.

All children had complete arrest of their cavities and "in no instance did this require more than ten weeks."[45] The oral hygiene of the children was in many cases very poor. The researchers also noted that "some of the children with arrest of caries did not use a toothbrush while away from the hospital."

# Lady May Mellanby &
# Dr. Weston A. Price

The systemic effects of food on cavities were also studied by two separate notable individuals in different parts of the world, around the same time, in the early to mid-1900s. Lady May Mellanby in Britain and Dr. Weston A. Price, from the United States.

## Lady May Mellanby

In Britain, Lady May Mellanby conducted extensive research on cavities in children, and is one of my idols! I can't help but be amazed by her accomplishments and research regarding systemic health and cavities, such a forward-thinking topic, at a time before women were even allowed to vote. As a woman dentist, I am grateful to Lady May Mellanby and all the other women who likely endured challenges beyond what I can even imagine so that women today do not need to.

Between 1917 and 1944, Lady May Mellanby had numerous publications in the *British Medical Journal*, the *British Dental Journal*, *The Lancet* and others about large-scale research studies involving dogs, as well as children's teeth and cavities.

For example, the *British Medical Journal* published a longitudinal study conducted by Lady May Mellanby with dentist, Helen Coumoulos involving nearly three thousand five-year-old children in London, England over a period of fifteen years.[46] The purpose of the study was to determine the effect, if any, of the government's wartime food policy on children's dental health. After the First World War, the British government started the "Cheap Milk Campaign," which provided all children with two-thirds of a pint of milk per day at either a reduced price or free of charge, depending on social status. In addition to the milk, children, infants and pregnant and lactating women were provided with cod liver oil, orange juice, and eggs. Also, calcium carbonate was added to bread and vitamins D2 and A were added to margarine.

At the onset of the experiment, 95% of the children had cavities, over 50% being classified as advanced cavities, with many children being completely edentulous (they had all their teeth extracted due to cavities).

After fifteen years, there was a drastic change in the oral health of the children. Only 6% of children had advanced cavities, and none were edentulous (with no teeth). Nearly 80% of the children still had cavities, but most of the cavities were small cavities.

Lady May Mellanby was an avid promoter of a diet high in fat-soluble vitamins and low in grains. She promoted the following nutritional protocol:

- An increased consumption of milk

- An increased consumption of eggs

- An increased consumption of foods high in 'calcifying factors'

- A decreased intake of bread, oatmeal and oatmeal preparations

- The addition of cod liver oil or some other source of vitamins D and A, especially the former

Lady May Mellanby advocated this nutritional protocol to pregnant mothers and children, as some of her studies were focused on the development of teeth, and she found that children had better-developed teeth when the mothers followed her prescribed nutritional protocol. (The teeth were studied microscopically and determined to be more or less calcified or dense than others).

## Dr. Weston A. Price

Another one of my idols, Dr. Weston A. Price made popular the idea that nutrition has a systemic effect on cavities and tooth development. Years ahead of himself, both with his respectful attitude towards aboriginal and native populations, which were called savages at the time, and with his dentistry, I aspire to do dentistry like he did. Helping people heal cavities using food that is beneficial for their systemic and oral health – that is just really awesome dentistry!

Dr. Weston A. Price was an American dentist who studied the dental (and overall) health of numerous indigenous races throughout the world, and found these groups of people to be almost completely free of cavities, and other modern degenerative diseases. His book, *Nutrition and Physical Degeneration*, originally published in 1939, is still very popular today and a highly interesting read. Dr. Price found that even though all of the groups of people he studied throughout the world had very different diets, there were some constant factors, such as a high intake of fat-soluble vitamins. In his dental office in Cleveland, Ohio, Dr. Price used nutrition to successfully remineralize his patient's cavities. The following is the lunch diet that he fed school-aged children who were fed their normal diet at home:[47]

- Tomato or orange juice

- Teaspoon of a mixture of equal parts very high-vitamin natural cod liver oil and a high-vitamin butter

- Pint of vegetable stew, always containing plenty of very yellow carrots, along with either bone marrow and fine cuts of tender meat, fish chowder or organs of animals

- Cooked fruit with very little sweetening

- Rolls made from freshly ground whole wheat, spread with high-vitamin butter. Wheat was ground fresh every day.

- Two glasses of fresh whole milk.

Dr. Weston Price also made note that on several occasions the children's teachers commented on the remarkable improvements the children experienced at school.

# A Brief Discussion of Some of the Aforementioned Foods

## Cod Liver Oil

Cod liver oil is a rich source of vitamins A and D, both of which have been implicated in cavity reduction.

## Vitamin D

Vitamin D has been correlated with cavities from its first discovery in 1918.[48] Edward Mellanby, husband of Lady May Mellanby, found that rickets, a bone deficiency, could be cured by a component in cod liver oil. Following this, there was an outpouring of research studies correlating the link between cavities and Vitamin D.[49,50,51,52,53,54]

Vitamin D regulates how much calcium and phosphorus is absorbed from food. Low levels of Vitamin D result in reduced calcium absorption. Having adequate calcium levels in the blood is so critical to our health that the body will do whatever is necessary to ensure good blood-calcium levels. When the parathyroid hormone detects low levels of calcium in the blood, it signals for calcium to be released from bony structures where calcium is ample, which include the skeleton and to a lesser degree, teeth. Thus, low levels of Vitamin D can result in calcium being moved from the teeth into the blood, where it is needed more.[55] Low levels of Vitamin D also mean there will be less calcium available in saliva for remineralization.

### Vitamin D & Magnesium

Vitamin D requires magnesium to be metabolized.[56,57] Teeth are frequently associated with calcium, but actually calcium and magnesium share equal importance in the body.[58] A significant amount of the body's magnesium is stored in bones and teeth.[59,60,61] Magnesium helps regulate the amount of calcium in the blood and inside cells, and too much calcium in inappropriate places can cause problems, such as symptoms of heart disease.[62,63]

# Vitamin A

Around the same time as the popularity of research linking vitamin D to cavities, many studies were done correlating vitamin A with cavities. The results were mixed, with some researchers showing a correlation while others did not.[64]

It is thought that vitamin A may be necessary for the proper development of dentin, and deficiency can lead to increased future risk of cavities. In 1980, a publication by *Archives of Oral Biology*, detailed an experiment during which animals were made vitamin A deficient at birth but then subsequently received adequate vitamin A. When exposed to *Strepto-coccus mutans* bacteria, the animals that had a history of vitamin A deficiency experienced significantly more cavities than the animals that were born with sufficient levels.[65]

Ever since it was popular to study the effects of vitamin A and D on cavities there was heavy debate about the validity of the claims. Currently this is still a topic of debate in modern dentistry.

# Milk

Milk has long been promoted by dentistry as being good for teeth. Lauric acid, found in milk, has been shown to prevent plaque formation and prevent demineralization of teeth.[66] Lauricidin, a component of lauric acid, has been found to be highly effective against Gram-positive bacteria (which includes *Steptococcus mutans*). When lauricidin is added to a cavity-promoting diet, there is increased ability to stop cavity formation.[67]

Lauric acid is found in cow's milk, goat's milk, human breast milk, and is also very plentiful in coconut. However, it is present in the fat of foods, and in reduced fat milk, lauric acid is also reduced.

Compared to other sugars, lactose, the sugar found in milk, caused the least reduction in dentin fluid flow, and was least likely to increase risk of cavities.

**Dentin Fluid Reduction:**

**Sucrose > Glucose > Lactose**

Lactose absorption into blood is slower than other sugars, so blood-glucose levels are less affected. Also, compared to other sugars, lactose causes the least amount of blood-phosphate changes, and blood-phosphate changes are associated with increased susceptibility to cavities. Additionally, lactose favors the absorption of minerals such as calcium and phosphorus.[68]

# A Note on Breast-Feeding

Although there are conflicting available studies, many studies indicate that breast-feeding does not increase incidence of cavities.[69,70] In fact, some studies show that breast-feeding is associated with increased protection to cavities in the present and future of teeth.[71] However, every dentist knows that many children do develop cavities while breast-feeding. I recommend uncovering and correcting the underlying issue of why the cavities are developing. Perhaps the child's digestion needs to be improved to allow for the proper assimilation of nutrients from the breast milk. Or perhaps the milk is sitting on the teeth all night. Remember lactose is a sugar, and while sleeping, many children (and adults) have dry, acidic mouths.

Sugar + Dry Acidic Mouth = Extensive Damage + Decay.

Also, ensuring that the breast-feeding mother is obtaining sufficient nutrients herself can be beneficial to both mother and child. For example women who are vitamin D deficient will pass along vitamin D deficient milk to their child.[72]

## Vitamin $K_2$

Vitamin $K_2$ is necessary for proper calcium uptake into the teeth (and bones).[73] Vitamin $K_2$ can be found in grass-fed animal products, such as meat, cheese, milk and eggs, as well as the traditional Japanese fermented food, natto, for a non-animal source.

Growing up I remember always looking at a magnet on the kitchen fridge in the shape of a cheese triangle with a bite taken out of it. It said "Cheese Puts the Bite on Cavities." Cheese can provide many benefits to naturally prevent and remineralize cavities. In addition to calcium, cheese from the raw milk of grass-fed animals can provide Vitamin $K_2$, Vitamin D, cavity-resisting bacteria and a variety of vitamins and minerals. Instead of finishing a meal with a sugary dessert, why not finish a meal like the French do with some delicious cheese? Test your mouth pH after — I bet you'll see that the cheese neutralizes it!

## Vitamin C

Current research confirms that vitamin C is correlated to a reduction in cavities, probably due to its antioxidant capabilities.[74]

## Conclusion

The body is designed have healthy teeth and to heal teeth when necessary. Given the opportunity, the body will gladly do its job. It is up to us to give it that opportunity. Diet is a major factor in cavity development and progression, and is an area that we have significant control of. Every day, multiple times a day, we consume foods that will either help our body protect our teeth or hinder our body's innate protective mechanisms. Let's make sure that we all help maximize our healing abilities by the choices we make right now, at the next bite of food.

# 12

# At the Modern Dental Office

"We need your help to bridge the cultural divide...from a treatment society to a prevention society. I commend the emphasis of this Call to Action on prevention."

*– Surgeon General's Report*[1]

I t is very important to see a dentist when you are interested in naturally preventing and remineralizing cavities (and when you aren't interested, as well!). I believe that diagnostic knowledge and abilities are undervalued in today's society, including that of dentists, and that the importance and complexity of a diagnosis is misunderstood. Diagnosing decay is complex and requires the assessment and analysis of many diagnostic tools that complement a dentist's knowledge and experience. Part of the process of diagnosing a cavity involves detecting the cavity, estimating its size and depth and degree of demineralization and making a decision about whether the cavity is active or arrested, and if active, how quickly it is progressing.[2] Dentists are the only healthcare providers that are able to diagnose cavities.

When you are interested in naturally preventing and remineralizing cavities, a dentist's diagnosis is absolutely critical, as it can result in earlier detection and therefore more realistic and successful remineralization of cavities, as well as serve as a basis for monitoring existing active and arrested cavities.

I highly recommend making use of the tremendous diagnostic knowledge dentists have acquired through education and experience. I also highly recommend making use of the amazing diagnostic tools and technologies that have recently become available in dental offices.

# Action Steps & Options

## Early Detection

Remember, it is far easier to remineralize a small cavity than a large one, and a dentist can diagnosis a small cavity before you are even aware of any changes in your mouth. When you see a dentist regularly, you will be notified of the very beginning signs of a cavity forming. This means a cavity will be diagnosed when it is very small, and likely localized to the enamel (incipient).

At this point your dentist will discuss with you your options and one of two decisions will be made:

# Option #1: Restore Cavity

The first option is to get the cavity restored or filled. Restoring very small cavities is sometimes called "minimally invasive dentistry." A significant benefit of minimally invasive dentistry is that you will have a very small restoration, and smaller restorations offer many benefits over large ones, such as increased longevity, decreased short- and long-term sensitivity, and less potential damage to the pulp. Another benefit of having the small cavity restored is that you do not have to focus on remineralization techniques or see your dentist for frequent monitoring. Perhaps time is an issue or some other life circumstances make it an inopportune time to focus on remineralizing the cavity. Although remineralization techniques are always and forever beneficial in preventing cavities, sometimes people only have time for the bare essentials.

## Option #2: Attempt Remineralization

The other option is to attempt to remineralize the cavity. If you take this option, you should see your dentist every three months for monitoring.[3]

**What to do if:**

If the cavity does not remineralize and progresses beyond the enamel, you should have a restoration completed immediately.[4] A cavity that progresses that much in three months is not only an actively progressing cavity, but likely a rapidly progressing cavity, and although your remineralization efforts have not been a waste of time, they have not been successful in arresting the cavity. In this case, have the cavity restored, and focus on remineralization techniques to slow down your rate of cavity progression before attempting to remineralize cavities.

**What to do if:**

If the cavity does not remineralize, and grows larger but is still very small and localized to the enamel, you can either choose to get a restoration (see Option #1) or continue to work on remineralizing. Continue with monitoring at your dentist's office every three months if you and your dentist decide that attempting to remineralize the cavity is still your best route of action.[5]

**What to do if:**

If the cavity becomes arrested and is remineralized, celebrate your success! Congratulations! You do not need to have the arrested cavity monitored every 3 months, although some people are more comfortable with frequent monitoring, which is obviously okay. Otherwise, you should have the arrested cavity monitored (as well as your other teeth) during the dentist's exam at your regular check-up appointments, which should be at least every year.[6]

## Treatment Options for Baby Teeth

Deciduous or "baby" teeth have different treatment options than adult or permanent teeth. Discuss these options with your dentist to see what is right for you and your family. If remineralization of a cavity on a deciduous tooth does not occur and the cavity grows, the deciduous tooth can be extracted, and little lasting damage will be incurred. An adult or permanent tooth that does not remineralize can result in significant lasting negative consequences, such as a root canal or extraction. For this reason, it can be appealing to attempt to remineralize baby teeth. However, remember children have a significantly higher risk of cavities than adults, and the cavities progress more rapidly. Attempting to remineralize tiny cavities in reasonable locations is a good idea for deciduous and permanent teeth, but if a cavity does not arrest in a baby tooth, it is highly likely that an infection will occur. An infection can present with pain or no pain, swelling in the gums around the tooth or pus. If any sign of infection appears around the baby tooth, the tooth should be immediately extracted. Stop working at remineralizing the cavity, cut your losses and get the tooth pulled. No amount of delay is acceptable to leave an infected baby tooth in a child's mouth. An infection or abscess that is left can cause permanent damage to the adult teeth located within the bone near the infected baby tooth. **Do Not Under Any Circumstances Leave an Infected Baby Tooth.**

# The Monitoring Process

## How to Know if a Cavity is Remineralized

An important distinction between active and arrested decay is determined by assessing whether the cavity is hard or soft. If the cavity is hard, it is remineralized, arrested, healed, hardened or however one wishes to say it. If the cavity is soft, it is an active cavity and is progressing either rapidly, slowly or somewhere in between.[7,8]

Of course, if you touch your finger to your tooth, whether there is an active cavity or not, it will always feel hard. Assessing the hardness or softness of a cavity must be done by a dentist, usually with a special dental instrument called an explorer. An explorer is a dental tool used to detect cavities and tartar, and for other aspects of dentistry and hygiene. It comes in different shapes and sizes, but always has a very sharp, thin tip, sort of like a needle or safety-pin tip. Touching an explorer on healthy tooth structure, including arrested decay, feels like touching a safety pin to your fingernail. Pushing really hard on your fingernail with a safety pin could damage your fingernail, but pushing really hard on healthy enamel with an explorer should not do any damage since enamel is the hardest substance in the body – harder than bone and certainly fingernails. Touching an explorer tip to active decay is sort of like touching a safety-pin tip into a raison or date. It is soft and sticky, or "leathery." Pushing hard with an explorer on a spot that is in the process of remineralizing can result in significant damage. The explorer is so sharp that it will break through any somewhat hardened tooth structure and result in a hole or cavity, properly called a cavitation in the tooth. Any remineralization that was achieved is lost, and remineralization will need to start over from the beginning, or else the cavity will progress.

The explorer is also capable of causing damage that results in more rapid progression of an existing active cavity. Once a cavity is fully remineralized, an explorer will not cause damage. There are some dental professionals who are advocates for eliminating the use of the explorer in diagnosing cavities. However, dental professionals are taught not to push hard on teeth with the explorer, and dentists know not to use force when diagnosing cavities. The explorer, when used properly, provides very valuable information to the dentist for the person interested in remineralizing their teeth and cavities. The explorer can aid in differentiating arrested and active decay, and help the dentist determine if a cavity has remineralized or not.[9,10,11]

**Explorer Pushed Excessively on Active Cavity = Cavity Progresses More Quickly**

**Explorer Pushed Excessively on Partially Arrested Cavity = Remineralized Areas Destroyed and Active Cavity Again**

**Explorer Pushed Excessively on Fully Arrested Cavity = No Problem**

Testing cavity hardness or softness with an explorer is a delicate endeavor. In fact, no part of the tooth should ever be touched with large amounts of pressure from the explorer, in case slight demineralization or remineralization is occurring. If no softness is felt using an explorer, there should be no additional force used, since the additional force may induce softness, especially in the grooves on the biting surfaces of teeth (occlusal surfaces).[12]

Do not under any circumstances try to assess the hardness of a cavity yourself. Do not use a safety pin, needle or dental explorer yourself. You can do some serious damage to your teeth. I am only discussing safety pins so you can be more educated about the process used at a dental office, not because I am suggesting you should do it yourself. You must see a dentist who has been trained to use an explorer to diagnose cavities. (Hygienists have been trained to use dental explorers for tartar detection.) The explorer may seem like a simple and straight forward tool, but it is capable of causing damage.

Sometimes decay is not visible and assessable when using an explorer. While an explorer can extend slightly further than the naked eye, there are many cavities that can't be assessed using the explorer, such as those occurring in between teeth (interproximal).

The best way to assess the activity of decay that is only visible in an X-ray is by taking additional X-rays to make sure the cavity is not growing. Using X-rays (properly called radiographs) is the gold standard way of monitoring decay, arrested or not, that is not visible to the naked eye. There are new technologies available in some dental offices that can detect and monitor some types of cavities without the use of radiation. Examples include lasers, quantitative light-induced fluorescence, electrical resistance and near-infrared technologies.

## Arrested Decay & X-Rays

Arrested decay will still show up in an X-ray.[13] Remember, the missing tooth structure does not grow back when a cavity is arrested (like a fingertip heals but does not grow back), and it is for this reason that arrested decay will still show up in an X-ray as a "hole." It is sometimes possible to see a faint radiopaque (lighter) layer on the most outward surface of an arrested cavity, but that is not always the case.[14] Radiopaque means the X-ray appears lighter or "whiter," and is indicative of a more dense area. Since the outer layer of an arrested cavity within dentin is usually lined with eburnated and sclerotic dentin, which is denser than regular dentin, this can very occasionally be seen in an X-ray, but it certainly should not be relied upon. Commonly, an arrested cavity will still appear to be radiolucent – or less porous on an X-ray, even though it has remineralized.[15] In these cases, arrested decay will appear the same as active decay in an X-ray. It is sort of like a scar.[16] This does not mean the area is any more likely to develop a cavity than the rest of the tooth (if the area is indeed arrested decay). Just like the scar I have on my leg from a dog bite when I was young, the skin is healed but it does not appear exactly as it did before the injury. But I still say that my skin is healed, and it is certainly no more likely to start bleeding than the rest of my skin.

Again, the X-ray will not show a completely absent cavity, rather it will show a scar of a cavity, if the cavity is arrested. An arrested decay scar and an active cavity will often appear the same.[17] The difference between the two is that the active cavity will grow and get bigger, while the arrested decay will not. If the presence of eburnated or sclerotic dentin is visible on the X-ray, consider that to be a bonus, because often it is not. For cavities that cannot be accessed by an explorer, the only way to know if the cavity is active or arrested is by monitoring its growth, or lack thereof. Even if it has grown a tiny amount, this is a sign of an active cavity. No growth means the cavity is arrested.

If the cavity is visible to the naked eye and/or accessible to a dental explorer your dentist will be able to tell you immediately whether the cavity is arrested and a cause for celebration, or if it is active and growing.

If the cavity is not visible to the naked eye and is only visible in an X-ray, the process of determining whether it is arrested or active is a lengthy one and your dentist won't be able to tell you immediately.[18]

Periodic X-rays will need to be taken, and if the cavity never grows then it can be confirmed as arrested. You will need to discuss with your dentist the frequency of these X-rays. Diagnostic technologies that do not use radiation may be used in addition to or in some cases instead of X-rays for monitoring arrested and active cavities.

## Pain

Pain is not a good indication of whether or not a tooth has remineralized. If you have pain from a cavity, it is quite likely because the cavity is so large it has reached the nerve and the nerve is infected. An infected nerve can result in an abscess in the bone surrounding the root of the tooth. This is like a pimple in the skin, which is often painful to touch. Except the skin is flexible and bone is not, and an abscess in bone is sometimes excruciatingly painful. A cavity that has grown to the point of nerve infection is clearly not arrested. Sometimes people say they do not want to do anything about their teeth or a cavity because they have no pain. However, waiting for pain to occur before doing something is setting yourself up for losing a tooth or having some major dental problems.

**Pain = Problem**

## Color of the Cavity

There are two common misconceptions regarding the color of a cavity. They are:

1. A dark-colored cavity is a bad sign.

2. A remineralized cavity reverses its color back to tooth-colored.

Both of these ideas are false. This is very good news for many people because it means that cavities they might have previously thought were active, growing cavities are actually arrested and healed. So often people come into my dental office pointing to a little brown spot they noticed on one of their teeth at home. Usually worried that it is a cavity, they are relieved to hear that it is arrested decay and does not require a filling. Of course, sometimes it is an active cavity, but more often than not I find myself telling people it is arrested. Every now and then, someone will choose to have the arrested decay restored because they don't like the look of the brown spot, especially if it is visible to others.

The brown color of a cavity is usually unrelated to its activity level (either progressing or arrested.) The color occurs because of extrinsic staining during a period of demineralization. A period of remineralization then follows and locks the extrinsic staining into the surface of the tooth.

Remember, demineralization of enamel is the removal of minerals from the tooth surface. Wherever the minerals were located, there is now nothing there, like tiny microscopic spaces in the enamel. Like Swiss cheese. Now let's say that someone with a demineralized spot on their tooth drinks some coffee, red wine, chaga mushroom tea or has some other staining food or drink. Those microscopic holes where their enamel is demineralized allow the staining substance to enter. Just like you could fill the holes of Swiss cheese. Now imagine that the tooth environment changes to one that promotes re-mineralization. This means the hydroxyapatite minerals are put back into the tooth. The minerals fill in the holes and the tooth surface is hard again, but this time there is some staining stuck within the tooth surface. It would be like putting the wrapper on the Swiss cheese, locking in whatever was put into the holes while the wrapper was off. Except unlike a cheese wrapper, the tooth surface cannot be removed (which is good!) and the stain is permanently stuck in the tooth. No amount of brushing or professional cleanings will remove the stain that is locked into the tooth. The only way the stain can be removed is by drilling it out, which is not necessary to do, unless the person wants to have the stain removed for cosmetic purposes.

Arrested decay stain is different than extrinsic staining that occurs without demineralization. Extrinsic staining without demineralization does not involve the incorporation of the stain into the structure of the tooth, and can be removed.

## Metals of Honor

I like to think of arrested decay brown spots (properly termed "brown spot lesions") as medals of honor. I know most people do not think of them as a good thing. People either think nothing of them or worry about them, as if they are going to become a cavity at any second. Brown spot lesions are a sign that cavities can heal, and if you have one or many, this means you healed your teeth and avoided one or many fillings. Sure they don't look that great, but the tooth is healthy and resilient and that is great news. If you want to restore a brown spot lesion, do so for cosmetic reasons, not because you are afraid it is going to become a sinister cavity in the future. Remember, once an area on a tooth is remineralized, it is often even more resistant to future decay, and that is regardless of whether it has had staining trapped in it or not. In fact, if a tooth goes through the demineralization and remineralization phases without any extrinsic staining occurring in between, it would be very challenging to know that those stages even occurred. Without extrinsic staining, one could have areas on their teeth demineralize and remineralize and not even realize it.

People seem to think that in order for a cavity to remineralize it must return to its original look and color. Not only does this not normally happen, but usually it is not even pos-

sible to do so. Relying on color change as an indicator of remineralization is not a good idea, and will usually result in dis-
appointment for no reason. Sometimes I see people frustrated
and upset because they want to remineralize a cavity and they
think their efforts are useless because the tooth won't change
color. Usually the tooth is already remineralized and has been
for a while, but the person didn't realize it. Remember the
color of the cavity does not indicate whether it is active or arrested. The softness or hardness is an indication of activity.
An active cavity is soft or sticky when touched with an explorer and an arrested cavity is rock hard when touched.

## Don't Be Fooled By Appearance

Paradoxically, often the worst-looking cavity is arrested and
the less sinister-looking cavity is active and progressing. According to *Sturdevant's Art & Science of Operative Dentistry*, the
most rapidly progressing cavities are lightest in color and slowly progressing cavities are often dark due to extrinsic staining
over time.[19]

Some teeth have a chalky-white appearance when they are
demineralized, and many people think chalky white is a nor-
mal-looking tooth, but in fact it can be the sign of active decay. Not all chalky-white spots are cavities, it can be caused by
other things, but chalky-white and soft is a sure sign of active
decay.

## Shiny & Healthy

Another subtle change in the appearance of a tooth or cavity is its shininess. A shiny spot, whether it is brown, tooth-colored or bright white is quite likely a healthy spot – either arrested decay or no decay. This is because when the tooth surface is loaded up with its minerals, it will shine and appear lustrous, whereas a tooth or spot on a tooth that is in a state of demineralization, with a Swiss cheese structure, will appear duller and lack luster. This is regardless of the actual color and presence of or lack of external staining on a tooth. For example, a remineralized tooth full of coffee staining will appear shinier than a demineralized bleached-white tooth.

Don't be disappointed by or fear brown spot lesions. Celebrate them as a great success in healing your teeth.

## No Need to Be Alone

Even though we are all in charge of our own health, including our dental health, there is no need to go about it alone. Utilizing the expertise of dentists and other dental professionals will give you even more power to achieve the mouth and health you desire.

# 13

## Final Words

Picture a day in the life of a tollbooth operator on the I-190, a busy highway in Niagara Falls, New York. Drivers from Canada who want to enter the United States at the border crossing and vice versa must pass through a toll and pay three dollars. There are countless ways for someone to pay their toll. They can pay in Canadian currency or American. Both ways to pay are correct. They can pay with a five-dollar biooll and get two dollars in return. They can pay three one-dollar American bills or three Canadian loonies. At this particular toll, the person can even pay one one-dollar American bill and two Canadian loonies or a Canadian toonie, the two-dollar coin. The person could pay three hundred pennies! Or the person could pay by credit card or prepaid toll coins. All of these ways and many more are acceptable and correct ways for someone to pay the toll.

Imagine that someone asks the tollbooth operator what the correct way to pay for the toll is. The toll-booth operator would probably reply that it doesn't matter as long as it equals three dollars, in American or Canadian currency. But the person insists on knowing the correct way to pay. What could the tollbooth operator possibly say? There is simply no one right answer. There are many correct ways to pay. There are also many incorrect ways to pay the toll, like using Monopoly money or giving any amount less than $3. It is not possible for the tollbooth operator to say the one correct way to pay because it does not exist. He or she may certainly have preferred ways for people to pay, like not with three hundred pennies, and drivers may certainly have their own preference for paying, like with a credit card, but the fact remains that as long as the necessary conditions are met for the toll payment, the vehicle will be granted passage through the toll, regardless of anyone's preferences. The key is that the necessary conditions are met.

Imagine now that someone wants to know what the correct way to prevent and remineralize cavities is? Just like it is impossible for the tollbooth operator to say the one and only correct way to pay for the toll, it is impossible to say the one and only correct way to prevent and remineralize cavities. There is no one correct way because there are many correct ways to successfully remineralize teeth. There are also many ways that result in unsuccessful remineralization of teeth, which is clearly evident from the statistic that over 90% of the population has had at least one cavity.

Some people have a preferred method or diet or technique that they follow and/or promote others to follow, just like the tollbooth operator and drivers do. And others have a different preferred way that they follow and/or promote others to follow. As long as the necessary conditions for remineralization of teeth are met, it doesn't matter what technique is followed, successful remineralization will occur. Likewise, if the necessary conditions for remineralization are not met, it doesn't matter what technique is followed, cavities will develop or progress and teeth will not be remineralized.

Some of the most expansive and deepest areas of remineralized and hardened cavities I have seen have been in homeless people, as well as recovering drug abusers. I see it as a testament to the remarkable healing abilities of the body to see the body heal after undergoing such harsh conditions. Don't get me wrong, some of the most expansive and deepest areas of active decay (requiring extractions) I have ever seen have also been in homeless people and people of addictions. The point I am making is that it does not matter what foods you eat, which techniques you do or do not follow, or how you choose to live your life, if you have the three-dollars for the toll, you will be granted passage, and if you have the necessary conditions for healthy teeth, you will successfully remineralize your teeth and cavities.

# Experience & Knowledge From My Father

When I graduated from dental school in 2008, I joined my father and brother at my father's dental office. I was able to see the real-life results of what I had learned in dental school about remineralization. I saw arrested decay in many shapes and sizes – tiny areas to huge spans; shallow and deep in various locations. I saw newly monitored areas and I also saw arrested decay that was being monitored since 1975, in some of my father's first dental patients. Any of my questions and concerns about the longevity of arrested decay were answered and relieved and I quickly realized that remineralized teeth and cavities can definitely outlast dental restorations.

After seeing the strength of remineralized teeth I understood why I had learned in dental school to promote prevention and remineralization; to monitor some areas of decay for a long time or short time, and to assess, evaluate and diagnose as a priority over being quick to draw the drill.

I learned that some sinister-looking cavities are harmless and some harmless-looking cavities are potential disasters. It became clear to me that a dentist's diagnosis is a complex undertaking and absolutely critical.

## My Hope for This Book

After I heard the crowd go wild in response to the popular health and wellness expert when he said he healed a cavity, I realized that not everyone is aware of the healing capabilities of teeth. I decided that I want to share my knowledge about teeth and cavities with others.

I am so grateful for the opportunity to see first-hand the remarkable healing abilities of the body every day when I look in people's mouths. I want everyone to know this amazingness that each and every one of us possesses!

My hope is that this book will help you find and create the necessary conditions so that you and your family can have the teeth you desire.

# Endnotes

# Chapter 1

[1] "Diagnosis and Management of Dental Caries Throughout Life," National Institutes of Health Consensus Development Conference Statement March 26-28, 2001, assessed Feb 19, 2015, http://consensus.nih.gov/2001/2001DentalCaries115html.htm.

[2] Roberson TM, Heymann HO, Swift EJ. *Sturdevant's Art & Science of Operative Dentistry*, 4th ed. (Chapel Hill, North Carolina: Mosby, Inc, 2002), 93.

[3] Roberson TM, Heymann HO, Swift EJ. *Sturdevant's Art & Science of Operative Dentistry*, 4th ed. (Chapel Hill, North Carolina: Mosby, Inc, 2002), 93-94.

[4] Roberson TM, Heymann HO, Swift EJ. *Sturdevant's Art & Science of Operative Dentistry*, 4th ed. (Chapel Hill, North Carolina: Mosby, Inc, 2002), 276.

[5] Steinman RR. The physiologic nature of caries susceptibility - Part III. J Alabama Dent Assn 67: 46-49, 1983.

[6] Carounanidy U, Sathyanarayanan R. Dental Caries - A Complete Changeover (Part 1). J Conserv Dent 12(2): 46-54, 2009.

[7] Roberson TM, Heymann HO, Swift EJ. *Sturdevant's Art & Science of Operative Dentistry*, 4th ed. (Chapel Hill, North Carolina: Mosby, Inc, 2002), 89-90.

[8] Roberson TM, Heymann HO, Swift EJ. *Sturdevant's Art & Science of Operative Dentistry*, 4th ed. (Chapel Hill, North Carolina: Mosby, Inc, 2002), 243.

[9] Hebling J, Pashley DH, Tjaderhane L, et al. Chlorhexidine arrests subclinical degradation of dentin hybrid layers in vivo. J Dent Res 84: 741-6, 2005.

[10] Carriho MR, Geraldeli S, Tay F, et al. In vivo preservation of the hybrid layer by chlorhexidine. J Dent Res 86: 529-33, 2007.

[11] Carriho MR, Carvalho RM, de Goes MF, et al. Chlorhexidine preserves dentin bond in vitro. J Dent Res 86: 90-94, 2007.

[12] Roberson TM, Heymann HO, Swift EJ. Sturdevant's *Art & Science of Operative Dentistry*, 4th ed. (Chapel Hill, North Carolina: Mosby, Inc, 2002), 30.

[13] Pashley DH. Clinical correlations of dentin structure and function. J Prosthet Dent 66(6): 777-781, 1991.

[14] Roberson TM, Heymann HO, Swift EJ. *Sturdevant's Art & Science of Operative Dentistry*, 4th ed. (Chapel Hill, North Carolina: Mosby, Inc, 2002), 144.

[15] Pashley DH. Clinical correlations of dentin structure and function. J Prosthet Dent 66(6):777-781, 1991.

[16] Roberson TM, Heymann HO, Swift EJ. *Sturdevant's Art & Science of Operative Dentistry*, 4th ed. (Chapel Hill, North Carolina: Mosby, Inc, 2002), 144-5.

[17] Casamassimo PS, Fields HW Jr, McTigue DJ, Nowak AJ. *Pediactric Dentistry Infancy through Adolescence* 4th ed. (St. Louis, Missouri: Elsevier Saunder, 2005), 530-531.

[18] Nathanson D, Lertpitayakun P, Lamkin MS et al. In vitro elution of leachable components from dental sealants. JADA 128: 1517, 1997.

[19] Fung EYK, Ewoldsen NO, St Germain HA, et al. Pharmacokinetics of bisphenol A released from a dental sealant. JADA 131:51, 2000.

[20] Roberson TM, Heymann HO, Swift EJ. *Sturdevant's Art & Science of Operative Dentistry*, 4th ed. (Chapel Hill, North Carolina: Mosby, Inc, 2002), 109.

# Chapter 2

[1] "Bisphenol A Facts," Canadian Dental Association, accessed Feb 11, 2015, http://www.cda-adc.ca/en/oral_health/faqs/bpa_faqs.asp#5.

[2] Roberson TM, Heymann HO, Swift EJ. *Sturdevant's Art & Science of Operative Dentistry*, 4th ed. (Chapel Hill, North Carolina: Mosby, Inc, 2002), 66.

[3] Kidd EAM, Fejerskov O. What Constitutes Dental Caries? Histopathology of Carious Enamel and Dentin Related to the Action of Cariogenic Biofilms. J Dent Res 83(Spec Iss C): C35-C38, 2004.

[4] Roberson TM, Heymann HO, Swift EJ. *Sturdevant's Art & Science of Operative Dentistry*, 4th ed. (Chapel Hill, North Carolina: Mosby, Inc, 2002), 94.

[5] Roberson TM, Heymann HO, Swift EJ. *Sturdevant's Art & Science of Operative Dentistry*, 4th ed. (Chapel Hill, North Carolina: Mosby, Inc, 2002), 90, 98, 424.

[6] Kidd EAM, Fejerskov O. What Constitutes Dental Caries? Histopathology of Carious Enamel and Dentin Related to the Action of Cariogenic Biofilms. J Dent Res 83(Spec Iss C): C35-C38, 2004.

[7] Roberson TM, Heymann HO, Swift EJ. (*Sturdevant's Art & Science of Operative Dentistry*, 4th ed. (Chapel Hill, North Carolina: Mosby, Inc, 2002), 89.

[8] Carounanidy U, Sathyanarayanan R. Dental Caries: A complete changeover (Part II) – Changeover in the diagnosis and prognosis. J Conserv Dent 12(3): 87–100, 2009.

[9] Carounanidy U, Sathyanarayanan R. Dental Caries: A complete changeover (Part II) – Changeover in the diagnosis and prognosis. J Conserv Dent 12(3): 87–100, 2009.

[10] Kidd EAM, Fejerskov O. What Constitutes Dental Caries? Histopathology of Carious Enamel and Dentin Related to the Action of Cariogenic Biofilms. J Dent Res 83(Spec Iss C): C35-C38, 2004.

[11] Roberson TM, Heymann HO, Swift EJ. *Sturdevant's Art & Science of Operative Dentistry*, 4th ed. (Chapel Hill, North Carolina: Mosby, Inc, 2002), 109.

[12] Roberson TM, Heymann HO, Swift EJ. *Sturdevant's Art & Science of Operative Dentistry*, 4th ed. (Chapel Hill, North Carolina: Mosby, Inc, 2002), 17.

[13] Fuller JL, Denehy GE, Schulein TM. *Concise Dental Anatomy and Morphology* 4th ed. (Iowa: University of Iowa, 2001), 11.

[14] Fuller JL, Denehy GE, Schulein TM. *Concise Dental Anatomy and Morphology* 4th ed. (Iowa: University of Iowa, 2001), 138.

[15] Fuller JL, Denehy GE, Schulein TM. *Concise Dental Anatomy and Morphology* 4th ed. (Iowa: University of Iowa, 2001), 11.

[16] Roberson TM, Heymann HO, Swift EJ. *Sturdevant's Art & Science of Operative Dentistry*, 4th ed. (Chapel Hill, North Carolina: Mosby, Inc, 2002), 22.

[17] Roberson TM, Heymann HO, Swift EJ. *Sturdevant's Art & Science of Operative Dentistry*, 4th ed. (Chapel Hill, North Carolina: Mosby, Inc, 2002), 23

[18] Roberson TM, Heymann HO, Swift EJ. *Sturdevant's Art & Science of Operative Dentistry*, 4th ed. (Chapel Hill, North Carolina: Mosby, Inc, 2002), 97, 276, 23.

[19] Kidd EAM, Fejerskov O. What Constitutes Dental Caries? Histopathology of Carious Enamel and Dentin Related to the Action of Cariogenic Biofilms. J Dent Res 83(Spec Iss C): C35-C38, 2004.

[20] Roberson TM, Heymann HO, Swift EJ. *Sturdevant's Art & Science of Operative Dentistry*, 4th ed. (Chapel Hill, North Carolina: Mosby, Inc, 2002), 22.

[21] Roberson TM, Heymann HO, Swift EJ. *Sturdevant's Art & Science of Operative Dentistry*, 4th ed. (Chapel Hill, North Carolina: Mosby, Inc, 2002), 26, 97, 276.

[22] Roberson TM, Heymann HO, Swift EJ. *Sturdevant's Art & Science of Operative Dentistry*, 4th ed. (Chapel Hill, North Carolina: Mosby, Inc, 2002), 97.

[23] Roberson TM, Heymann HO, Swift EJ. *Sturdevant's Art & Science of Operative Dentistry*, 4th ed. (Chapel Hill, North Carolina: Mosby, Inc, 2002), 98.

[24] Roberson TM, Heymann HO, Swift EJ. *Sturdevant's Art & Science of Operative Dentistry*, 4th ed. (Chapel Hill, North Carolina: Mosby, Inc, 2002), 97, 276, 424.

[25] Kidd EAM, Fejerskov O. What Constitutes Dental Caries? Histopathology of Carious Enamel and Dentin Related to the Action of Cariogenic Biofilms. J Dent Res 83(Spec Iss C): C35-C38, 2004.

[26] Manji F, Fejerskov O, Nagelkerke NJD, et al. A random effects model for some epidemiological features of dental caries. Community Dent Oral Epidemiol 19: 324-28, 1991.

[27] Hojo S, Komatsu M, Okauda R, et al. Acid Profiles and pH of Carious Dentin in Active and Arrested Lesions. J Dent Res 73(12): 1853-1857, 1994.

[28] Kidd EAM, Fejerskov O. What Constitutes Dental Caries? Histopathology of Carious Enamel and Dentin Related to the Action of Cariogenic Biofilms. J Dent Res 83(Spec Iss C): C35-C38, 2004.

[29] Roberson TM, Heymann HO, Swift EJ. *Sturdevant's Art & Science of Operative Dentistry*, 4th ed. (Chapel Hill, North Carolina: Mosby, Inc, 2002), 89-90.

[30] Kidd EAM, Fejerskov O. What Constitutes Dental Caries? Histopathology of Carious Enamel and Dentin Related to the Action of Cariogenic Biofilms. J Dent Res 83(Spec Iss C): C35-C38, 2004.

[31] Rosenstiel SF, Land MF, Fujimoto J. *Contemporary Fixed Prosethodontics* 3rd ed. (St. Louis, Missouri: Mosby, Inc, 2001), 64.

[32] Roberson TM, Heymann HO, Swift EJ. *Sturdevant's Art & Science of Operative Dentistry*, 4th ed. (Chapel Hill, North Carolina: Mosby, Inc, 2002), 97, 276, 22.

[33] White JM, Eakle WS. Rationale and treatment approach in minimally invasive dentistry. J Am Dent Assoc 131 Suppl: 13S-19S, 2000.

[34] Kidd EAM, Fejerskov O. What Constitutes Dental Caries? Histopathology of Carious Enamel and Dentin Related to the Action of Cariogenic Biofilms. J Dent Res 83(Spec Iss C): C35-C38, 2004.

[35] Larmas M, Dental Caries Seen from the Pulpal Side: a Non-traditional Approach. J Dent Res 82(4): 253-6, 2003.

[36] Kidd EAM, Fejerskov O. What Constitutes Dental Caries? Histopathology of Carious Enamel and Dentin Related to the Action of Cariogenic Biofilms. J Dent Res 83(Spec Iss C): C35-C38, 2004.

[37] Kidd EAM, Fejerskov O. What Constitutes Dental Caries? Histopathology of Carious Enamel and Dentin Related to the Action of Cariogenic Biofilms. J Dent Res 83(Spec Iss C): C35-C38, 2004.

[38] Roberson TM, Heymann HO, Swift EJ. *Sturdevant's Art & Science of Operative Dentistry*, 4th ed. (Chapel Hill, North Carolina: Mosby, Inc, 2002), 92.

[39] Parfitt GJ. The speed of development of the carious cavity. Br Dent J 100: 204-207, 1956.

[40] Roberson TM, Heymann HO, Swift EJ. *Sturdevant's Art & Science of Operative Dentistry*, 4th ed. (Chapel Hill, North Carolina: Mosby, Inc, 2002), 92.

[41] Holmen L, Thylstrup A, Artun J. Clinical and histological features observed during arrestment of active enamel carious lesions in vivo. Caries Res 21: 546-54, 1987.

[42] Holmen L, Thylstrup A, Artun J. Surface changes during the arrest of active enamel carious lesions in vivo. A scanning electron microscopic study. Acta Odontol Scand 45: 383-390, 1987.

[43] Roberson TM, Heymann HO, Swift EJ. *Sturdevant's Art & Science of Operative Dentistry*, 4th ed. (Chapel Hill, North Carolina: Mosby, Inc, 2002), 109.

# Chapter 3

[1] Roberson TM, Heymann HO, Swift EJ. *Sturdevant's Art & Science of Operative Dentistry*, 4th ed. (Chapel Hill, North Carolina: Mosby, Inc, 2002), 103.

[2] Roberson TM, Heymann HO, Swift EJ. *Sturdevant's Art & Science of Operative Dentistry*, 4th ed. (Chapel Hill, North Carolina: Mosby, Inc, 2002), 101.

[3] Imfield T. Dental erosion. Definition, classification and links. Eur J Oral Sci 104(Pt 2): 151-5, 1996.

[4] Wu CD. Grape Products and Oral Health. J Nutr 139(9): S1818-23, 2009.

# Chapter 4

[1] Roberson TM, Heymann HO, Swift EJ. *Sturdevant's Art & Science of Operative Dentistry*, 4th ed. (Chapel Hill, North Carolina: Mosby, Inc, 2002), 109.

[2] Dawes C. What is the critical pH and why does a tooth dissolve in acid? J Can Dent Assoc 69(11):722-4, 2003.

[3] Ricketts RM. The Cranial Base and Soft Structures in Cleft Palate Speech and Breathing. Plast Reconstr Surg 14(1): 47-61, 1954.

[4] Lind MG, Lundell BPW. Tonsillar hyperplasia in children. Arch Otolaryngol 108: 650–654, 1982.

[5] Guilleminault C, Korobkin R, Winkle R. A review of 50 children with obstructive sleep apnea syndrome. Lung 159: 275–287, 1981.

[6] Brouillette R, Hanson D, David R, et al. A diagnostic approach to suspected obstructive sleep apnea in children. J Pediatr 105: 10–14, 1984.

[7] Anders TF, Carskadon MA, Dement WC, et al. Sleep habits of children and the identification of pathologically sleepy children. Child Psychiatr Hum Dev 9: 56–63, 1978.

[8] Kravath RE, Pollak CP, Borowiecki B. Hypoventilation during sleep in children who have lymphoid airway obstruction treated by nasopharyngeal tube and T and A. Pediatrics 59: 865–871, 1977.

[9] Noonan JA. Reversible cor pulmonale due to hypertrophied tonsils and adenoids: studies in two cases. Circulation 31/32: 164, 1965.

[10] Weissbluth M, Davis AT, Poncher J, et al. Signs of airway obstruction during sleep and behavioral, developmental and academic problems. J Dev Behav Pediatr 4: 119–121, 1983.

[11] Carskadon MA, Pueschel SM, Millman RP. Sleep-disordered breathing and behavior in three risk groups: preliminary findings from parental reports. Childs Nerv Syst 9(8): 452-7, 1993.

[12] Hugo FN, Hilgert JB, Corso S, et al. Association of chronic stress, depression symptoms and cortisol with low saliva flow in a sample of south-Brazilians aged 50 years and older. Gerodontology 25(1): 18-25, 2008.

[13] Tremblay M, Brisson B, Gaudet D. Association between salivary pH and metabolic syndrome in women: a cross-sectional study BMC Oral Health **12**: 40, 2012.

[14] Morgan BL, Kuyatt BL, Flink J. Effects of hypothyroidism on the DNA, carbohydrate, soluble protein and sialic acid contents of rat submandibular glands. J Oral Pathol 14(1): 37-41, 1985.

[15] "Saliva Testing Good Practice Good Sense," GC Corporation, accessed Feb 11, 2015, http://www.scribd.com/doc/60266795/Saliva-Test-Brochure#scribd.

[16] Ramesh G, Nagarajappa R, Madhusudan AS, et al. Estimation of salivary and tongue coating pH on chewing household herbal leaves: A randomized controlled trial. Anc Sci Life 32(2): 69–75, 2012.

[17] Hancock PJ, Epstein JB, Sadler GR. Oral and Dental Management Related to Radiation Therapy for Head and Neck Cancer. J Can Dent Assoc 69(9): 585–90, 2003.

[18] Amaechi BT, Higham SM. Dental erosion: possible approaches to prevention and control J Dent Mar 33(3): 243-52, 2005.

[19] Hancock PJ, Epstein JB, Robins Sadler G. Oral and Dental Management Related to Radiation Therapy for Head and Neck Cancer J Can Dent Assoc 69(9): 585–90, 2003.

[20] Konig D, Muser K, Dickhuth H-H, et al. Effect of a supplement rich in alkaline minerals on acid-base balance in humans Nutr J 8: 23, 2009.

[21] Roberson TM, Heymann HO, Swift EJ. *Sturdevant's Art & Science of Operative Dentistry*, 4th ed. (Chapel Hill, North Carolina: Mosby, Inc, 2002), 89.

[22] Severinghaus JW. Simple, accurate equations for human blood O2 dissociation computations. J Appl Physiol Respir Environ Exerc Physiol 46(3):599-602, 1979.

[23] Carounanidy U, Sathyanarayanan R. Dental Caries - A Complete Changeover (Part 1). J Conserv Dent 12(2): 46-54, 2009.

[24] Beers MH, Fletcher AJ, Jones TV, et al. *The Merck Manual of Medical Information* 2nd ed. (Whitehouse Station: Merck Research Laboratories, 2003), 932.

[25] Beers MH, Fletcher AJ, Jones TV, et al. *The Merck Manual of Medical Information* 2nd ed. (Whitehouse Station: Merck Research Laboratories, 2003), 932.

[26] Beers MH, Fletcher AJ, Jones TV, et al. *The Merck Manual of Medical Information* 2nd ed. (Whitehouse Station: Merck Research Laboratories, 2003), 932.

[27] Beers MH, Fletcher AJ, Jones TV, et al. *The Merck Manual of Medical Information* 2nd ed. (Whitehouse Station: Merck Research Laboratories, 2003), 932.

# Chapter 5

[1] Roberson TM, Heymann HO, Swift EJ. *Sturdevant's Art & Science of Operative Dentistry*, 4th ed. (Chapel Hill, North Carolina: Mosby, Inc, 2002), 68.

[2] Newman HN. The relation between plaque and dental caries. J Roy Soc Med 79(14): 1-5, 1986

[3] Roberson TM, Heymann HO, Swift EJ. *Sturdevant's Art & Science of Operative Dentistry*, 4th ed. (Chapel Hill, North Carolina: Mosby, Inc, 2002), 67.

[4] Lazarchik, DA, Frazier KB. Dental erosion and acid reflux disease: An overview. Gen Dent 57(2): 151-6, 2009.

[5] Roberson TM, Heymann HO, Swift EJ. *Sturdevant's Art & Science of Operative Dentistry*, 4th ed. (Chapel Hill, North Carolina: Mosby, Inc, 2002), 67.

[6] Roberson TM, Heymann HO, Swift EJ. *Sturdevant's Art & Science of Operative Dentistry*, 4th ed. (Chapel Hill, North Carolina: Mosby, Inc, 2002), 67.

[7] Alaluusua S, Renkonen OV. *Streptococcus mutans* establishment and dental caries experience in children from 2 to 4 years old. Scand J Dent Res.91(6): 453-7, 1983.

[8] Kristoffersson K, Gröndahl HG, Bratthall D. The more *Streptococcus mutans*, the more caries on approximal surfaces. J Dent Res. 64(1): 58-61, 1985.

[9] Bowen WH. Food components and caries. Adv Dent Res 8(2): 215-20, 1994.

[10] Milgrom P, Zeo DT, Tanzer JM. An Examination of the Advances in Science and Technology of Prevention of Tooth Decay in Young Children Since the Surgeon General's Report on Oral Health. Academic Pediatrics 9(6): 404-409, 2009.

[11] Simratvir M, Singh N, Chopra S, et al. Efficacy of 10% povidone iodine in children affected with early childhood caries: an in vivo study. J Clin Pediatr Dent 34(3): 233–8, 2010.

[12] Lopez L, Berkowitz R, Zlotnik H, et al. Topical antimicrobial therapy in the prevention of early childhood caries. Pediatr Dent 21(1): 9–11, 1999.

[13] Tam A, Shemesh M, Wormser U, et al. Effect of different iodine formulations on the expression and activity of Streptococcus mutans glucosyltransferase and fructosyltransferase in biofilm and planktonic environments. J Antimicrob Chemoth 57(5): 865–71, 2006.

[14] Amin MS, Harrison RL, Benton TS. Effect of povidone-iodine on Streptococcus mutans in children with extensive dental caries. Pediatr Dent 26(1): 5-10, 2004.

[15] Kashket S, DePaola DP. Cheese consumption and the development and progression of dental caries. Nutr Rev 60(4): 97-103, 2002.

[16] Rivero-Cruz JF,, Zhu M, Kinghorn AD et al. Antimicrobial constituents of Thompson seedless raisins (Vitis vinifera) against selected oral pathogens. Phytochem Lett. 2008; 1:151-4.

[17] Benjamin S, Roshni, Thomas SS, et al. Grape Seed Extract as a Potential Remineralizing Agent: A Comparative in vitro Study. J Contemp Dent Pract 13(4): 425-30, 2012.

[18] Ferrazzano GF, Amato I, Ignenito A, et al. Plant Polyphenols and Their Anti-Cariogenic Properties: A Review. Molecules 16: 1486-507, 2011.

[19] Packer L, Colman C. *The Antioxidant Miracle* (MA: John Wiley & Sons, Inc, 1999), 118.

[20] Cai L, Wu CD. Compounds from Syzgium aromaticum possessing growth inhibitory activity against oral pathogens. J Nat Prod. 1996; 59:987-90.

[21] Dole V, Kharat P, Ali Khan M. Zinc Oxide Eugenol - A Multidisciplinary Approach in Dentistry. J Cont Med A Dent 1(1): 4-7 , 2013.

[22] *"Ceanothus americanus,"* Wikimedia Foundation, Inc, accessed Feb 11, 2015, http://en.wikipedia.org/wiki/Ceanothus_americanus

[23] Li XC, Cai L, Wu CD. Antimicrobial compounds from Ceanothus americanus against oral pathogens. Phytochemistry. 1997; 46:97-102.

[24] Cai L, Wei GX, van der Bijl P, et al. Namibian chewing stick, Diospyros lycidoides, contains antibacterial compounds against oral pathogens. J Agric Food Chem. 2000; 48:909-14.

[25] Li XC, van der Bijl P, Wu CD. Binaphthalenone glycosides from African chewing sticks, Diospyros lycidides. J Nat Prod. 1998; 61:817-20.

[26] Hwang BY, Roberts SK, Chadwick LR et al. Antimicrobial constituents from goldenseal (the Rhizomes of Hydrastis canadensis) against selected oral pathogens. Planta Med. 2003; 69:623-7.

[27] Chadwick LRW, Wu CD, Kinghorn AD. Isolation of alkaloids from goldenseal (Hydrastis canadensis rhizomes) using pH zone-refining countercurrent chromatography. J Liq Chromataogr Rel Technol. 2001; 24:2445-53.

[28] He J, Chen L, Heber D, et al. Antibacterial compounds from Glycyrrhiza uralensis. J Nat Prod 69(1): 121–4, 2006.

[29] Mäkinen KK, Mäkinen PL, Pape HR Jr, et al. Conclusion and review of the Michigan Xylitol Programme (1986-1995) for the prevention of dental caries. Int Dent J 46(1): 22-34, 1996.

[30] Roberson TM, Heymann HO, Swift EJ. *Sturdevant's Art & Science of Operative Dentistry*, 4th ed. (Chapel Hill, North Carolina: Mosby, Inc, 2002), 67.

[31] Loesche WJ. Role of *Streptococcus mutans* in human dental decay. Microbiol Rev 50: 353-380, 1986.

[32] Carounanidy U, Sathyanarayanan R. Dental Caries - A Complete Changeover (Part 1). J Conserv Dent 12(2): 46-54, 2009.) (Marsh PD. Microbial ecology of dental plaque and its significance in health and disease. Adv Dent Res 8(2): 263-71, 1994.

[33] Roberson TM, Heymann HO, Swift EJ. *Sturdevant's Art & Science of Operative Dentistry*, 4th ed. (Chapel Hill, North Carolina: Mosby, Inc, 2002), 91

[34] Roberson T, Heymann HO, Swift EJ. *Sturdevant's Art & Science of Operative Dentistry*, 4th ed. (Chapel Hill, North Carolina: Mosby, Inc, 2002), 87.

[35] "Colonisation," Memidex, accessed Feb 11, 2015, http://www.memidex.com/colonisation.

[36] Roberson TM, Heymann HO, Swift EJ. *Sturdevant's Art & Science of Operative Dentistry*, 4th ed. (Chapel Hill, North Carolina: Mosby, Inc, 2002), 68-80.

[37] Roberson TM, Heymann HO, Swift EJ. *Sturdevant's Art & Science of Operative Dentistry*, 4th ed. (Chapel Hill, North Carolina: Mosby, Inc, 2002), 87.

[38] Kidd EAM, Fejerskov O. What Constitutes Dental Caries? Histopathology of Carious Enamel and Dentin Related to the Action of Cariogenic Biofilms. J Dent Res 83(Spec Iss C): C35-C38, 2004.

[39] Roberson TM, Heymann HO, Swift EJ. *Sturdevant's Art & Science of Operative Dentistry*, 4th ed. (Chapel Hill, North Carolina: Mosby, Inc, 2002), 89)

[40] Kjersti A, Ma J, Antony KM, et al. The Placenta Harbors a Unique Microbiome. Sci Transl Med 6(237): 237ra65, 2014.

[41] Roberson TM, Heymann HO, Swift EJ. *Sturdevant's Art & Science of Operative Dentistry*, 4th ed. (Chapel Hill, North Carolina: Mosby, Inc, 2002), 75.

[42] Jett BD, Gilmore MS: The growth inhibitory effect of the Enterococcus faecalis bacteriocin encoded by pAD1 extends to the oral streptococci, J Dent Res 69(10):1640-1645, 1990.

[43] Loyola-Rodriguiez JP et al: Purification and properties of extracellular mutacin, a bacteriocin from Streptoccus sobrinus, J Gen Microbiol 138(pt2):269-274, 1992.

[44] Koll-Klais P, Mändar R, Leibur E, Marcotte H, Hammarström L. Mikelsaar M. Oral lactobacilli in chronic periodontitis and periodontal health: species composition and antimicrobial activity. Oral Microbiol Immunol 20(6): 354-61, 2005.

[45] Krasse P, Carlsson B, Dahl C, Paulsson A, Nilsson A, Sinkiewicz G. Decreased gum bleeding and reduced gingivitis by the probiotic Lactobacillus reuteri. Swed Dent J 30(2): 55-60, 2006.

[46] Kang MS, Kim BG, Chung J, Lee HC, Oh JS. Inhibitory effect of Weissella cibaria isolates on the production of volatile sulphur compounds. J Clin Periodontol. 2006;33(3):226-32, 2006.

[47] Sookkhee S, Chulasiri M, Prachyabrued W. Lactic acid bacteria from healthy oral cavity of Thai volunteers: inhibition of oral pathogens. J Appl Microbiol 90(2): 172-9, 2001.

[48] Bonifait L, Chandad F, Grenier D. Probiotics for oral health: myth or reality? J Can Dent Assoc 75(8): 585-90, 2009.

[49] Madigan MT, Martinko JM, Parker J. *Brock Biology of Microorganisms* 10th ed. (New Jersey: Pearson Education, Inc, 2003), 732,953.

[50] Meurman JH, Antila H, Salminen S. Recovery of Lactobacillus strain GG (ATCC 53103) from saliva of healthy volunteers after consumption of yoghurt prepared with the bacterium. Microbiol Ecol Health Dis 7(6): 295-8, 1994.

[51] Yli-Knuuttila H, Snäll J, Kari K, Meurman JH. Colonization of Lactobacillus rhamnosus GG in the oral cavity. Oral Microbiol Immunol 21(2): 129-31, 2006.

[52] Ooshima T, Yasufuku Y, Izumitani A: Effect of mutacin administration on *Streptococcus mutans*-induced dental caries in rats, Microbiol Immunol 29(12):1163-1173, 1985.

[53] Campbell-McBride N. *Gut and Psychology Syndrome: Natural Treatment for Autism, ADD/ADHD, Dyslexia, Dyspraxia, Depression, Schizophrenia* 2nd ed. (Medinform Publishing, 2010).

[54] Roberson TM, Heymann HO, Swift EJ. *Sturdevant's Art & Science of Operative Dentistry*, 4th ed. (Chapel Hill, North Carolina: Mosby, Inc, 2002), 75,78.

[55] Ooshima T, Yasufuku Y, Izumitani A: Effect of mutacin administration on *Streptococcus mutans*-induced dental caries in rats, Microbiol Immunol 29(12):1163-1173, 1985.

[56] Madigan MT, Martinko JM, Parker J. *Brock Biology of Microorganisms* 10th ed. (New Jersey: Pearson Education, Inc, 2003), 403.

[57] Roberson TM, Heymann HO, Swift EJ. *Sturdevant's Art & Science of Operative Dentistry*, 4th ed. (Chapel Hill, North Carolina: Mosby, Inc, 2002), 67.

[58] Nase L, Hatakka K, Savilahti E, et al. Effect of Long-Term Consumption of a Probiotic Bacterium, Lactobacillus rhamnosus GG, in Milk on Dental Caries and Caries Risk in Children. Caries Res 35: 412-20, 2001.

[59] Roberson TM, Heymann HO, Swift EJ. *Sturdevant's Art & Science of Operative Dentistry*, 4th ed. (Chapel Hill, North Carolina: Mosby, Inc, 2002), 78, 101.

[60] Carounanidy U, Sathyanarayanan R. Dental Caries - A Complete Changeover (Part 1). J Conserv Dent 12(2): 46-54, 2009.

[61] Marsh PD. Microbial ecology of dental plaque and its significance in health and disease. Adv Dent Res 8(2): 263-71, 1994.

[62] Roberson TM, Heymann HO, Swift EJ. *Sturdevant's Art & Science of Operative Dentistry*, 4th ed. (Chapel Hill, North Carolina: Mosby, Inc, 2002), 76.

[63] Roberson TM, Heymann HO, Swift EJ. *Sturdevant's Art & Science of Operative Dentistry*, 4th ed. (Chapel Hill, North Carolina: Mosby, Inc, 2002), 110.

# Chapter 6

[1] Roberson TM, Heymann HO, Swift EJ. *Sturdevant's Art & Science of Operative Dentistry*, 4th ed. (Chapel Hill, North Carolina: Mosby, Inc, 2002), 103.

[2] Su N, Marek CL, Ching V, et al. "Caries Prevention for Patients with Dry Mouth." J Can Dent Assoc 77: b85, 2011.

[3] Roberson TM, Heymann HO, Swift EJ. *Sturdevant's Art & Science of Operative Dentistry*, 4th ed. (Chapel Hill, North Carolina: Mosby, Inc, 2002), 89.

[4] "Saliva Testing Good Practice Good Sense," GC Corporation, accessed Feb 11, 2015, http://www.scribd.com/doc/60266795/Saliva-Test-Brochure#scribd.

[5] "Saliva Testing Good Practice Good Sense," GC Corporation, accessed Feb 11, 2015, http://www.scribd.com/doc/60266795/Saliva-Test-Brochure#scribd.

[6] "Saliva Testing Good Practice Good Sense," GC Corporation, accessed Feb 11, 2015, http://www.scribd.com/doc/60266795/Saliva-Test-Brochure#scribd.

[7] "Saliva Testing Good Practice Good Sense," GC Corporation, accessed Feb 11, 2015, http://www.scribd.com/doc/60266795/Saliva-Test-Brochure#scribd.

[8] Dawes C. What is the critical pH and why does a tooth dissolve in acid? J Can Dent Assoc 69(11):722-4, 2003.

[9] Scully C. Drug effects on salivary glands: dry mouth. Oral Dis 9(4):165-76, 2003.

[10] Osterberg T, Landahl S, Hedegård BJ Salivary flow, saliva, pH and buffering capacity in 70-year-old men and women. Correlation to dental health, dryness in the mouth, disease and drug treatment. Oral Rehabil 11(2): 157-70, 1984.

[11] Scully C. Drug effects on salivary glands: dry mouth. Oral Dis 9(4):165-76, 2003.

[12] Scully C. Drug effects on salivary glands: dry mouth. Oral Dis 9(4):165-76, 2003.

[13] Carlson GW. The salivary glands. Embryology, anatomy, and surgical applications. Surg Clin North Am 80: 261–273, 2000.

[14] Scully C. Drug effects on salivary glands: dry mouth. Oral Dis 9(4):165-76, 2003.

[15] "Saliva Testing Good Practice Good Sense," GC Corporation, accessed Feb 11, 2015, http://www.scribd.com/doc/60266795/Saliva-Test-Brochure#scribd.

[16] Scully C. Drug effects on salivary glands: dry mouth. Oral Dis 9(4):165-76, 2003.

[17] Wardrop RW[1], Hailes J, Burger H, et al. Oral discomfort at menopause. Oral Surg Oral Med Oral Pathol.67(5): 535-40, 1989.

[18] Hancock PJ, Epstein JB, Sadler GR. Oral and Dental Management Related to Radiation Therapy for Head and Neck Cancer. J Can Dent Assoc 69(9): 585–90, 2003.

[19] Wardrop RW[1], Hailes J, Burger H, et al. Oral discomfort at menopause. Oral Surg Oral Med Oral Pathol.67(5): 535-40, 1989

[20] Agha-Hosseini F, Mirzaii-Dizgah I, Mansourian A, et al. Relationship of stimulated saliva 17beta-estradiol and oral dryness feeling in menopause Maturitas. 20;62(2):197-9, 2009.

[21] Scully C. Drug effects on salivary glands: dry mouth. Oral Dis 9(4):165-76, 2003.

[22] Carounanidy U, Sathyanarayanan R. Dental Caries - A Complete Changeover (Part 1). J Conserv Dent 12(2): 46-54, 2009.

[23] Hancock PJ, Epstein JB, Sadler GR. Oral and Dental Management Related to Radiation Therapy for Head and Neck Cancer. J Can Dent Assoc 69(9): 585–90, 2003.

# Chapter 7

[1] Roberson TM, Heymann HO, Swift EJ. *Sturdevant's Art & Science of Operative Dentistry*, 4th ed. (Chapel Hill, North Carolina: Mosby, Inc, 2002), 110.

[2] Chaussain-Miller C, Fioretti F, Goldberg M et al. The Role of Matrix Metalloproteinases (MMPs) in Human Caries. J Dent Res 85(1): 22-32, 2006.

[3] Hideaki H, Woessner J Jr. Matrix Metalloproteinases. J Biol Chem 274: 21491-4, 1999.

[4] Chaussain-Miller C, Fioretti F, Goldberg M et al. The Role of Matrix Metalloproteinases (MMPs) in Human Caries. J Dent Res 85(1): 22-32, 2006.

[5] Chaussain-Miller C, Fioretti F, Goldberg M et al. The Role of Matrix Metalloproteinases (MMPs) in Human Caries. J Dent Res 85(1): 22-32, 2006.

[6] Gibson D, Cullen B, Legerstee R, et al. MMPs made easy. Wounds International 1(1), 2009, http://woundsinternational.com/made-easys/mmps-made-easy.

[7] Chaussain-Miller C, Fioretti F, Goldberg M et al. The Role of Matrix Metalloproteinases (MMPs) in Human Caries. J Dent Res 85(1): 22-32, 2006.

[8] Chaussain-Miller C, Fioretti F, Goldberg M et al. The Role of Matrix Metalloproteinases (MMPs) in Human Caries. J Dent Res 85(1): 22-32, 2006.

[9] Palosaari H, Pennington CJ, Larmas M et al. Expression profile of matrix metalloproteinases (MMPs) and tissue inhibitors of MMPs in mature human odontoblasts and pulp tissue. Eur J Oral Sci 111: 117-27, 2003.

[10] van Strijp AJ, Jansen DC, DeGroot J, et al. Host-derived proteinases and degradation of dentine collagen in situ. Caries Res 37: 58-65, 2003.

[11] Goldberg M, Septier D, Bourd K, et al. Immunohistochemical localization of MMP-2, MMP-9, TIMP-1, and TIMP-2 in the forming rat incisor. Connect Tissue Res 44: 143-53, 2003.

[12] Bourd-Boittin K, Septier D, Hall R, et al. Immunolocalization of enamelysin (matrix metalloproteinase-20) in the forming rat incisor. J Histochem Cytochem 52: 437-45, 2004.

[13] Chaussain-Miller C, Fioretti F, Goldberg M et al. The Role of Matrix Metalloproteinases (MMPs) in Human Caries. J Dent Res 85(1): 22-32, 2006.

[14] Farges JC, Romeas A, Melin M, et al. TGF-beta 1 induces accumulation of dendritic cells in the odontoblast layer. J Dent Res 82: 652-6, 2003.

[15] Mu D, Cambier S, Fjellbirkeland L, et al. The integrin alpha(v)beta(8) mediates epithelial homeostasis through MTI-MMP-dependent activation of TGF-beta1. J Cell Biol 157: 493-507.

[16] Chaussain-Miller C, Fioretti F, Goldberg M et al. The Role of Matrix Metalloproteinases (MMPs) in Human Caries. J Dent Res 85(1): 22-32, 2006.

[17] Roberson TM, Heymann HO, Swift EJ. *Sturdevant's Art & Science of Operative Dentistry*, 4th ed. (Chapel Hill, North Carolina: Mosby, Inc, 2002), 96.

[18] Chaussain-Miller C, Fioretti F, Goldberg M et al. The Role of Matrix Metalloproteinases (MMPs) in Human Caries. J Dent Res 85(1): 22-32, 2006.

[19] Bourd-Boittin K, Fridman R, Fanchon S, et al. Matrix metalloproteinase inhibition impairs the processing, formation and mineralization of dental tissues during mouse molar development. Exp Cell Res 304: 493-505, 2005.

[20] Goldberg M, Septier D, Bourd K, et al. Immunohistochemical localization of MMP-2, MMP-9, TIMP-1, and TIMP-2 in the forming rat incisor. Connect Tissue Res 44: 143-53, 2003.

[21] Katz S, Park KK, Palenik CJ. In-vitro root surface caries studies. J Oral Med 42: 40-8, 1987.

[22] van Strijp AJ, van Steenbergen TJ, de Graaff J, et al. Bacterial colonization and degradation of demineralized dentin matrix in situ. Caries Res 28: 21-7, 1994.

[23] van Strijp AJ, van Steenbergen TJ, ten Cate JM. Bacterial colonization of mineralized and completely demineralized dentine in situ. Caries Res 31: 349-55, 1997.

[24] Kawasaki K, Featherstone JD. Effects of collagenase on root demineralization. J Dent Res 76: 588-595, 1997.

[25] Tjaderhane L, Aapistie O, Larjava H, et al. The Activation and Function of Host Matrix Metalloproteinases in Dentin Matrix Breakdown in Caries Lesions. J Dent Res 77(8): 1622-29, 1998.

[26] Dumas J, Hurion N, Weil R, et al. Collagenase in mineralized tissues of human teeth. FEBS Lett 187: 51-55, 1985.

[27] Dung SZ, Gregory RL, Li Y, et al. Effect of lactic acid and proteolytic enzymes on the release of organic matrix components from human teeth. Caries Res 29: 483-9, 1995.

[28] Baker AH, Edwards DR, Murphy G. Metalloproteinase inhibitors: biological actions and therapeutic opportunities. J Cell Sci 115: 3719-27, 2002.

[29] Gunja-Smith Z, Woessner JF Jr. Activation of cartilage stromelysin-1 at acid pH and its relation to enzyme pH optimum and osterarthritis. Agents Actions 40: 228-31, 1993.

[30] Davis GE. Identification of an abundant latent 94-kDa gelatin-degrading metalloproteinase in human saliva which is activated by acid exposure: implications for a role in digestion of collagenous proteins. Arch Biochem Biophys 286: 551-4, 1001.

[31] Chaussain-Miller C, Fioretti F, Goldberg M et al. The Role of Matrix Metalloproteinases (MMPs) in Human Caries. J Dent Res 85(1): 22-32, 2006.

[32] Amy Sang Q-X, Jin Y, Newcomer RG, et al. Matrix Metalloproteinase Inhibitors as Prospective Agents for the Prevention and Treatment of Cardiovascular and Neoplastic Diseases. Curr Top Med Chem 6: 289-316, 2006.

[33] Rasmussen HS, McCann PP. Matrix metalloproteinase inhibition as a novel anticancer strategy: a review with special focus on batimastat and marimastat. Pharmocol Ther 75: 69-75, 1997.

[34] Evans JD, Stark A, Johnson CD, et al. A phase II trial of marimastat in advanced pancreatic cancer. Br J Cancer 85: 1865-70, 2001.

[35] Wojtowicz-Praga SM, Dickson RB, Hawkins MJ. Matrix metalloproteinase inhibitors. Invest New Drugs 15: 61-75, 1997.

[36] Bramhall SR, Schulz J, Nemunaitis J, et al. A double-blind placebo-controlled, randomized study comparing gemcitabine and marimastat with gemcitabine and placebo at first line therapy in patients with advanced pancreatic cancer. Br J Cancer 87: 161-7, 2002.

[37] Overall CM, Lopez-Otin C. Strategies for MMP inhibition in cancer: innovations for the post-trial era. Nat Rev Cancer 2: 657-72, 2002.

[38] Gu Y, Dee CM, Shen J. Interaction of free radicals, matrix metalloproteinases and caveolin-1 impacts blood-brain barrier permeability. Front Biosci 3: 1216-31, 2011.

[39] Overall CM, Lopez-Otin C. Strategies for MMP inhibition in cancer: innovations for the post-trial era. Nat Rev Cancer 2: 657-72, 2002.

[40] Kato MT, Leite AL, Hannas AR, et al. Gels Containing MMP Inhibitors Prevent Dental Erosion in situ. J Dent Res 89: 468-72, 2010.

[41] Tjaderhane L, Sulkala M, Sorsa T, et al. The effect of MMP inhibitor metastat on fissure caries progression in rats. Ann NY Acad Sci 878: 686-8, 1999.

[42] Sulkala M, Wahlgren J, Larmas M, et al. The effects of MMP inhibitors on human salivary MMP activity and caries progression in rats. J Dent Res 80: 1545-9, 2001.

[43] Hebling J, Pashley DH, Tjaderhane L, et al. Chlorhexidine arrests subclinical degradation of dentin hybrid layers in vivo. J Dent Res 84: 741-6, 2005.

[44] Carriho MR, Geraldeli S, Tay F, et al. In vivo preservation of the hybrid layer by chlorhexidine. J Dent Res 86: 529-33, 2007.

[45] Carriho MR, Carvalho RM, de Goes MF, et al. Chlorhexidine preserves dentin bond in vitro. J Dent Res 86: 90-94, 2007.

[46] Kut C, Assoumou A, Dridi M, et al. Morphometric analysis of human gingival elastic fibres degradation by human leukocyte elastase protective effect of avocado and soybean unsaponifiables (ASU). Pathol Biol 46: 571-6, 1998.

[47] "Lupinus albus," Wikipedia, assessed Feb 11, 2015, http://en.m.wikipedia.org/wiki/Lupinus_albus

[48] Gaultier F, Foucault-Bertaud A, Lamy E, et al. Effects of a vegetable extract from *Lupinus albus* (LU105) on the production of matrix metalloproteinases (MMP1, MMP2, MMP9) and tissue inhibitor of metalloproteinases (TIMP1, TIMP2) by human gingival fibroblasts in culture. Clin Oral Investig 7: 198-205, 2003.

[49] Lord RS, Bralley JA. *Laboratory Evaluations for Integrative and Functional Medicine* 2nd ed. (Duluth, Georgia: Metametrix Institute, 2008), 275.

[50] Huet E, Cauchard JH, Berton A, et al. Inhibition of plasmin-mediated prostromelysin-1 activation by interaction of long chain unsaturated fatty acids with kringle 5. Biochem Pharmacol 67: 643-4, 2004.

[51] Berton A, Rigot V, Huet E, et al. Invovlement of fibronectin type II repeats in the efficient inhibition of gelatinases A and B by long-chain unsaturated fatty acids. J Biol Chem 276: 20458-65, 2001.

[52] Muktar H, Ahmad N. Green tea in chemoprevention of cancer. Toxicol Sci 52: 111-7, 1999.

[53] Sartor L, Pezzato E, Dell'Aica I, et al. Inhibition of matrix-proteases by poly-phenols: chemical insights for anti-inflammatory and anti-invasion drug design. Biochem Pharmacol 64: 229-37, 2002.

[54] Demeule M, Brossard M, Page M, et al. Matrix metalloproteinases inhibition by green tea catechins. Biochim Biophys Acta 1478: 51-60, 2000.

[55] Garbisa S, Sartor L, Biggin S, et al. Tumor gelatinases and invasion inhibited by the green tea flavanol epigallocatechin-3-gallate. Cancer 91: 822-32, 2001.

[56] Chaussain-Miller C, Fioretti F, Goldberg M et al. The Role of Matrix Metal-loproteinases (MMPs) in Human Caries. J Dent Res 85(1): 22-32, 2006.

[57] Yoneda S[1], Suzuki KT. Detoxification of mercury by selenium by binding of equimolar Hg-Se complex to a specific plasma protein Toxicol Appl Pharmacol 143(2):274-80, 1997.

[58] Packer L, Colman C. *The Antioxidant Miracle* (MA: John Wiley & Sons, Inc, 1999), 142.

[59] Visse R, Nagase H. Matrix metalloproteinases and tissue inhibitors of metal-loproteinases: structure, function, and biochemistry. Circ Res 92: 827-9, 2003.

[60] Devasagayam TPA, Tilak JC, Boloor KK, et al. Free Radicals and Antioxi-dants in Human Health: Current Status and Future Prospects. J Assoc Physi-cians India 52: 794-804, 2004.

[61] Nagase H, Woessner JF Jr. Matrix Metalloproteinases. J Biol Chem 274: 21491-4, 1999.

[62] Gu Y, Dee CM, Shen J. Interaction of free radicals, matrix metalloproteinases and caveolin-1 impacts blood-brain barrier permeability. Front Biosci 3: 1216-31, 2011.

[63] Amy Sang Q-X, Jin Y, Newcomer RG, et al. Matrix Metalloproteinase Inhibitors as Prospective Agents for the Prevention and Treatment of Cardiovascular and Neoplastic Diseases. Curr Top Med Chem 6: 289-316, 2006.

[64] Liu KJ, Rosenberg GA. Matrix metalloproteinases and free radicals in cerebral ischemia. Free Radical Bio Med 39(1): 71–80, 2005.

[65] Machlin LJ, Bendich A. Free radical tissue damage: protective role of antioxidant nutrients. FASEB J 1(6):441-5, 1987.

[66] Avsar A, Darka O, Topaloglu B, et al. Association of passive smoking with caries and related salivary biomarkers in young children. Arch Oral Biol 53(10): 969-74, 2008.

[67] Freeman BA, Crapo JD. Biology of disease: free radicals and tissue injury. Lab Invest 47(5): 412-26, 1982.

[68] Machlin LJ, Bendich A. Free radical tissue damage: protective role of antioxidant nutrients. FASEB J 1(6):441-5, 1987.

[69] Freeman BA, Crapo JD. Biology of disease: free radicals and tissue injury. Lab Invest 47(5): 412-26, 1982.

[70] Liu J, Mori A. Stress, Aging, and Brain Oxidative Damage. Neurochem Res 24(11): 1479-97, 1999.

[71] Machlin LJ, Bendich A. Free radical tissue damage: protective role of antioxidant nutrients. FASEB J 1(6):441-5, 1987.

[72] Manuel y Keenoy B, Moorken G, Vertommen J, et al. Magnesium status and parameters of the oxidant-antioxidant balance in patients with chronic fatigue: effects of supplementation with magnesium. J Am Coll Nutr 19(3): 374-82, 2000.

[73] Albano E. Alcohol, oxidative stress and free radical damage. P Nutr Soc 65(3): 278-90, 2006.

[74] Muriel P. Role of Free Radicals in Liver Diseases. Hepatol Int 3: 526-36, 2009.

[75] Packer L, Colman C. *The Antioxidant Miracle* (MA: John Wiley & Sons, Inc, 1999), 107.

[76] Ji LL, Leichtweis S. Exercise and oxidative stress: Sources of free radicals and their impact on antioxidant systems AGE 20(2): 91-106, 1997.

[77] Sies H. *Antioxidants in Disease, Mechanisms and Therapy*. (New York: Academic Press, 1996).

[78] Scoditti E1, Calabriso N, Massaro M, et al. Mediterranean diet polyphenols reduce inflammatory angiogenesis through MMP-9 and COX-2 inhibition in human vascular endothelial cells: a potentially protective mechanism in atherosclerotic vascular disease and cancer. Arch Biochem Biophys 527(2):81-9, 2012.

[79] Benjamin S, Roshni, Thomas SS, et al. Grape Seed Extract as a Potential Remineralizing Agent: A Comparative *in vitro* Study. J Contemp Dent Pract 2012;13(4):425-430.

[80] Xie Q, Bedran-Ryssi AK, Wu CD. *In vitro* remineralization effects of grape seed extract on artificial root caries. J Dent 36: 900-06, 2008.

# Chapter 8

[1] Steinman RR, Leonora J. *Dentinal Fluid Transport*. (Loma Linda, California: The Loma Linda University Press, 2004), 119.

[2] Wu CD. Grape Products and Oral Health. J Nutr 139(9): S1818-23, 2009.

[3] Lui, FT. Effect of Estrogen, Thyroxin, and Their Combination on Dental Caries and Salivary Glands in Ovariectomized and Intact Female Rats. J Dent Res 46(3): 471-7, 1967.

[4] Bixler D, Muhler JC. The Relation of Thyroid Gland Activity to the Incidence of Dental Caries in the Rat. J Dent Res 36(6):880-2, 1957.

[5] Haldi J, Wynn W, Law MI. Relationship between Thyroid Function and Resistance to Dental Caries. J Dent Res 41(2): 398-404, 1962.

[6] Muhler JC, Shafer WG. Experimental Dental caries, IV. The Effect of Feeding Desiccated Thyroid and Thuouracil on Dental Caries in Rats. Science 119(3098): 687-9, 1954.

[7] Carbone DF, Sweeney EA, Shaw JJ. The comparative influence of thyroid imbalance and limited body weight gain on submandibular gland weight, the protein components of saliva and dental caries in the rat. Arch Oral Biol 11(8): 781-92, 1966.

[8] Bixler D, Muhler JC. The Relation of Systemic Fluoride and Thyroid Gland Activity to the Incidence of Dental Caries in the Rat. J Dent Res 36(2): 304-306, 1957.

[9] Muhler JC, Bixler D, Shafer WG. Effect of Replacement Therapy on Dental Caries Experience of Radiothyroidectomized Rats. Exp Biol Med 93(2): 328-30, 1956.

[10] Leese GP, Flynn RV, Jung RT et al. Increasing prevalence and incidence of thyroid disease in Tayside, Scotland: the Thyroid Epidemiology Audit and Research Study (TEARS). J Clin Endocrinol 68(2): 311-16, 2008.

[11] Flynn RWV, MacDonald M, Morris AD et al. The Thyroid Epidemiology, Audit, and Research Study: Thyroid Dysfunction in the General Population. J Clin Endocr Metab 89(8): 3879-84, 2004.

[12] "General Information/Press Room," American Thyroid Association, assessed Feb 11, 2015, www.thyroid.org/media-main/about-hypothyroidism/.

[13] Cooper GM. *The Cell: A Molecular Approach* 2nd ed. (Sunderland, MA: Sinauer Associates, 2000).

[14] Morgan BL, Kuyatt BL, Flink J. Effects of hypothyroidism on the DNA, carbohydrate, soluble protein and sialic acid contents of rat submandibular glands. J Oral Pathol 14(1): 37-41, 1985.

[15] Bardow A[1], Moe D, Nyvad B, et al. The buffer capacity and buffer systems of human whole saliva measured without loss of $CO2$. Arch Oral Biol 45(1):1-12, 2000.

[16] Beers MH, Fletcher AJ, Jones TV, et al. *The Merck Manual of Medical Information* 2nd ed. (Whitehouse Station: Merck Research Laboratories, 2003), 901.

[17] Awawdeh L, Lundy FT, Shaw C, et al. Quantitative analysis of substance P, neurkinin A, calcitonin gene-related peptide in pulp tissue from painful and healthy human teeth. International Endodontic Journal 35(1): 30-36, 2002.

[18] Beers MH, Fletcher AJ, Jones TV, et al. *The Merck Manual of Medical Information* 2nd ed. (Whitehouse Station: Merck Research Laboratories, 2003), 953.

[19] Beers MH, Fletcher AJ, Jones TV, et al. *The Merck Manual of Medical Information* 2nd ed. (Whitehouse Station: Merck Research Laboratories, 2003), 953-4.

[20] Christ-Crain M, Meier C, Guglielmetti M, et al. Elevated C-reactive protein and homocysteine values: cardiovascular risk factors in hypothyroidism? A cross-sectional and a double-blind, placebo-controlled trial Atherosclerosis 166(2): 379-86, 2003.

[21] Saito T, Murakami M, et al. Association Between Alveolar Bone Los and Elevated Serum C-Reactive Protein in Japanese Men. J Periodontol 74: 1741-6, 2003.

[22] Iwamoto Y, Nishimura F, et al. Antimicrobial Periodontal Treatment Decreases Serum C-Reactive Protein, Tumor Necrosis Factor-Alpha, But Not Adiponectin Levels in Patients with Chronic Periodontitis. J Periodontol 74: 1231-6, 2003.

[23] Mattila K, Vesanen M, et al. Effect of treating Periodontitis on C-reactive protein levels: a pilot study. BMC Infectious Diseases 2: 30, 2002.

[24] Tuter G, Kurtis B, Serdar M. Evaluation of Gingival Crevicular Fluid and Serum Levels on High-Sensitivity C-Reactive Protein in Chronic Periodontitis Patients With or Without Coronary Artery Disease. J Periodontol 78(12): 2319-24, 2007.

[25] Zhu YS, Yen PM, Chin WW et al. Estrogen and thyroid hormone interaction on regulation of gene expression. PNAS 93(22): 12587-92, 1996.

[26] "NCHS Health E-Stat Iodine Level, United States, (2000)," Centers for Disease Control and Prevention, assessed Feb 11, 2015, www.cdc.gov/nchs/data/hestat/iodine.htm.

[27] Gibson RS. *Principles of Nutritional Assessment* 2nd ed. (Oxford, New York: Oxford University Press Inc, 2005), 759.

[28] Hollowell JG, Staehling NW, Hannon WH, et al. Iodine Nutrition in the United States. Trends and Public Health Implications: Iodine Excretion Data from National Health and Nutrition Examination Surveys I and III (1971-1974 and 1988-1994). J Clin Endocr Metab 83(10): 3401-8, 2013.

[29] Dadachova E, Carrasco N. The Na/I symporter (NIS): imaging and therapeutic applications. Semin Nucl Med 34(1): 23-31, 2004.

[30] Jhiang SM[1], Cho JY, Ryu KY, et al. An immunohistochemical study of Na+/I- symporter in human thyroid tissues and salivary gland tissues. Endocrinology139(10): 4416-9, 1998.

[31] Spitzweg C, Joba W, Eisenmenger W, et al. Analysis of Human Sodium Iodide Symporter Gene Expression in Extrathyroidal Tissues and Cloning of Its Complementary Deoxyribonucleic Acids from Salivary Gland, Mammary Gland, and Gastric Mucosa. J Clin Endocr Metab 83(5): 1746-51, 1998.

[32] Spitzweg C, Joba W, Eisenmenger W, et al. Analysis of Human Sodium Iodide Symporter Gene Expression in Extrathyroidal Tissues and Cloning of Its Complementary Deoxyribonucleic Acids from Salivary Gland, Mammary Gland, and Gastric Mucosa. J Clin Endocr Metab 83(5): 1746-51, 1998.

[33] Spitzweg C, Joba W, Schriever K, et al. Analysis of human sodium iodide symporter immunoreactivity in human exocrine glands. Clin Endocrinol Metab. 84(11):4178-84, 1999.

[34] "NCHS Health E-Stat Iodine Level, United States, (2000),"Centers for Disease Control and Prevention, assessed Feb 11, 2015, www.cdc.gov/nchs/data/hestat/iodine.htm.

[35] Teng W, Shan Z, Teng X, et al. Effect of Iodine Intake on Thyroid Diseases in China. N Engl J Med 354(26): 2783-93, 2006.

[36] Dunn JT. What's happening to our iodine? J Clin Endocrinol Metab 83(10):3398-400, 1998.

[37] Dunn JT. What's happening to our iodine? J Clin Endocrinol Metab 83(10):3398-400, 1998.

[38] "Supplements & Herbs: Iodine," DrWeil.com, accessed Feb 22, 2015, http://www.drweil.com/drw/u/ART02872/iodine.html.

[39] Vobecky M, Babicky A. Effect of enhanced bromide intake on the concentration ratio I/Br in the rat thyroid gland. Biol Trace Elem Res 43-45: 509-16, 1994.

[40] van Leeuwen FXR, Hanemaaijer R, Loeber JG. The effect of sodium bromide on thyroid function. Arch Toxicol 12: 93-97, 1988.

[41] Velicky J, Titlbach M, Duskova J et al. Potassium bromide and the thyroid gland of the rat: morphology and immunohistochemistry, RIA and INAA analysis. Ann Anat 179(5):421-31, 1997.

[42] Galletti PM, Joyet G. Effect of fluorine on thyroidal iodine metabolism in hyperthyroidism. J Clin Endocr Metab 18(10): 1102-10, 1958.

[43] Anderson DL. Determination of Bromine in Regulated Foods with a Field-Portable X-Ray Fluorescence Analyzer. J AOAC Int 92(2): 502-10, 2009.

[44] "Facts about Bromine," Centers for Disease Control and Prevention, assessed Feb 15, 2015, http://emergency.cdc.gov/agent/bromine/basics/facts.asp.

[45] Richardson SD, DeMarini DM, Koqevinas M. What's in the Pool? A Comprehensive Identification of Disinfection By-Products and Assessment of Mutagenicity of Chlorinated and Brominated Swimming Pool Water. Environ Health Perspect 118(11): 1523-30, 2010.

[46] Yuita K. Overview and Dynamics of Iodine and Bromine in the Environment. JARQ 28: 100-11, 1994.

[47] Turner DL. Determination of Brominated Vegetable Oil Concentrations in Soft Drinks Using a Specific Ion Electrode. J Food Sci 37(5): 791-2, 1972.

[48] "Brominated vegetable oil," Wikipedia, assessed Feb 11, 2015, http://en.m.wikipedia.org/wiki/Brominated_vegetable_oil.

[49] "Flame retardant of hexabromodiphenylalkane, heptabromodiphenylalkane, and octabromodiphenylalkane which has a broad melting point range; flammable polymer and flame retardant," US Patent 6117371 A, assessed Feb 15, 2015, http://www.google.com/patents/US6117371.

[50] Lukacs JR, Largaespada LL. Explaining sex differences in dental caries prevalence: Saliva, hormones, and "life-history" etiologies. Am J Hum Biol 18(4): 540-555, 2006.

[51] Lukacs JR. Fertility and Agriculture Accentuate Sex Differences in Dental Caries Rates. Curr Anthropol 49(5): 901-14, 2008.

[52] Lukacs JR, Largaespada LL. Explaining sex differences in dental caries prevalence: Saliva, hormones, and "life-history" etiologies. Am J Hum Biol 18(4): 540-555, 2006.

[53] "Dental Caries (Tooth Decay) in Adults (Age 20 to 64)," National Institute of Dental and Craniofacial Research, assessed Feb 11, 2015, http://www.nidcr.nih.gov/DataStatistics/FindDataByTopic/DentalCaries/DentalCariesAdults20to64.htm.

[54] Liu FTY, Lofgen R, Hoots I. Effect of Steroid Hormones on Dental Caries and Salivary Glands in female Rats. J Dent Res 45:1236, 1966.

[55] Liu FTY. Infulence of Some Steroid Contraceptives on Incidence of Dental Caries and Changes in Salivary Glands in Female Rats. J Dent Res 47:1047-1055, 1968.

[56] Lui FTY, Lin HS. Effect of Some Contraceptive Steroids on Growth and Development of Salivary Glands and Incidence of Dental Caries in Female Rats. J Dent Res 48(3): 477-82, 1969.

[57] Shafer WG, Muhler JC. Effect of Gonadectomy and Sex Hormones on the Structure of the Rat Salivary Gland. J Dent Res 32: 262-268, 1953.

[58] Shafer WG, Muhler JC. Experimental Dental Caries: III. The Effect of Estradiol and Diethylstillbestrol on Dental Caries, Fluorine Metabolism, and the Salivary Glands of Intact and Gonadectomized Rats. J Dent Res 33: 842-848, 1954.

[59] Muhler JC, Shafer WG. Experimental Dental Caries: VII. The Effect of Various Androgens and Estrogens on Dental Caries in the Rat. J Dent Res 34: 661-665, 1955.

[60] Lui FT. Effect of Estrone and Estriol on Salivary Glands and Dental Caries in Female Rats. Proc Soc Exp Biol Med 124: 591-595, 1967.

[61] Lui FTY, Lin HS. Effect of the Contraceptive Steroids Norethynodrel and Mestranol on Dental Caries Activity in Young Adult Female Rats. J Dent Res 52(4): 753-7, 1973.

[62] Lui FTY, Lin HS, Zullo T. Effect of Graded Doses of Estradiol Benzoate on Dental Caries and Salivary Glands in Female Rats. J Dent Res 48(3):485, 1969.

[63] Lui, FT. Effect of Estrogen, Thyroxin, and Their Combination on Dental Caries and Salivary Glands in Ovariectomized and Intact Female Rats. J Dent Res 46(3): 471-7, 1967.

[64] Liu FTY. Infulence of Some Steroid Contraceptives on Incidence of Dental Caries and Changes in Salivary Glands in Female Rats. J Dent Res 47:1047-1055, 1968.

[65] Valimaa H, Savolainen S, Soukka T, et al. Estrogen receptor-beta is the predominant estrogen receptor subtype in human oral epithelium and salivary glands. J Endocrinol 180: 55-62, 2004.

[66] Valimaa H, Savolainen S, Soukka T, et al. Estrogen receptor-beta is the predominant estrogen receptor subtype in human oral epithelium and salivary glands. J Endocrinol 180: 55-62, 2004.

[67] Abraham GE, Maroulis GB. Effect of exogenous estrogen on serum pregnenolone, cortisol, and androgens in postmenopausal women. Obstet Gynecol 45(3): 271-4, 1975.

[68] Hietala EL, Larmas M. The effect of ovariectomy and high-sucrose diet on dentine formation and caries in growing rats. Arch Oral Biol. 39(11): 973-8, 1994.

[69] Hietala EL, Larmas M. The effect of ovariectomy on dentinal apposition and caries in adult animals. Acta Odont Scand 50(6): 337-43, 1992.

[70] Cebi S, Stephen KW. Caries prevalence and oral contraception. Community Dent Oral Epidemiol 7(3): 183-4, 1979.

[71] Cebi S, Stephen KW. Caries prevalence and oral contraception. Community Dent Oral Epidemiol 7(3): 183-4, 1979.

[72] Northrup C. Women's Bodies, Women's Wisdom. (United States: Random House, Inc, 2010), 521-585.

[73] Muhler JC. Experimental Dental Caries: VII. The Effect of Various Androgens and Estrogens on Dental Caries in the Rat. J Dent Res 34(5): 661-665, 1955.

[74] Steinman RR, Jardinge MG. The effect of pyridoxine and injected carbohydrate on the incidence of caries, dentinal circulation related to diet. J Dent Res 37(5): 874-9, 1958.

[75] Davis DL, Bradiow HL, Wolff M, et al. Medical Hypothesis: Xenoestrogens As Preventable Causes of Breast Cancer. Environmental Health Perspectives 101(5): 372-77, 1993.

[76] Davis DL, Bradiow HL, Wolff M, et al. Medical Hypothesis: Xenoestrogens As Preventable Causes of Breast Cancer. Environmental Health Perspectives 101(5): 372-77, 1993.

[77] "Indole-3-carbinol," Wikipedia, assessed Feb 11, 2015, http://en.m.wikipedia.org/wiki/Indole-3-carbinol.

[78] Smith AJ, Phipps WR, Thomas W. The Effects of Aerobic Exercise on Estrogen Metabolism in Healthy Premenopausal Women. Cancer Epidemiol Biomarkers Prev 22: 756, 2013.

[79] Davis DL, Bradiow HL, Wolff M, et al. Medical Hypothesis: Xenoestrogens As Preventable Causes of Breast Cancer. Environmental Health Perspectives 101(5): 372-77, 1993.

[80] Steinmetz R[1], Mitchner NA, Grant A, et al. The xenoestrogen bisphenol A induces growth, differentiation, and c-fos gene expression in the female reproductive tract.

Endocrinology 139(6):2741-7, 1998.

[81] C A Harris, P Henttu, M G Parker, et al. The estrogenic activity of phthalate esters in vitro. Environ Health Perspect105(8): 802–811, 1997.

[82] Osborne MP, Karmali RA, Hershcopf H, et al. Omega-3 Fatty Acids: Modulation of Estrogen Metabolism and Potential for Breast Cancer Prevention. Cancer Invest 6(5): 629-31, 1988.

[83] Meissner HO, Mrozikiewicz P, Bobkiewicz-Kozlowska T, et al. Hormone-Balancing Effect of Pre-Gelatinized Organic Maca (*Lepidium peruvianum* Chacon): (I) Biochemical and Pharmacodynamic Study on Maca using Clinical Laboratory Model on Ovariectomized Rats. Int J Biomed Sci 2(3): 260–72, 2006.

[84] Chlebowski RT, Hendrix SL, Langer RD, et al. Influence of Estrogen Plus Progestin on Breast Cancer and Mammography in Healthy Postmenopausal Women. JAMA 2003 June, 289(24): 3243-53.

[85] Schairer C, Lubin J, Troisi R, et al. Menopausal estrogen and estrogen-progestin replacement therapy and breast cancer risk. JAMA 2000 Jan, 283(4): 485-491.

# Chapter 9

[1]Steinman RR, Leonora J. *Dentinal Fluid Transport.* (Loma Linda, California: The Loma Linda University Press, 2004), 32.

[2] Roberson TM, Heymann HO, Swift EJ. *Sturdevant's Art & Science of Operative Dentistry*, 4th ed. (Chapel Hill, North Carolina: Mosby, Inc, 2002), 30.

[3] Roberson TM, Heymann HO, Swift EJ. *Sturdevant's Art & Science of Operative Dentistry*, 4th ed. (Chapel Hill, North Carolina: Mosby, Inc, 2002), 30.

[4] Roberson TM, Heymann HO, Swift EJ. *Sturdevant's Art & Science of Operative Dentistry*, 4th ed. (Chapel Hill, North Carolina: Mosby, Inc, 2002), 30.

[5] Steinman RR, Leonora J. Relationship of Fluid Transport Through the Dentin to the Incidence of Dental Caries. J Dent Res 50(6): 1536-42, 1971.

[6] Steinman RR, Leonora J, Tieche J-M. Susceptibility to dental caries. Aust Dent J 24(4): 222-4, 1979.

[7] Leonora J, Tieche J-M, Steinman RR. Stimulation of Intradentinal Dye Penetration by Feeding in the Rat. Archs oral Biol. 38(9): 763-69, 1993.

[8] Steinman RR, Leonora J. Acidogenic Potential of Cariogenic and Noncariogenic Diets in the Rat. 54(3): 578-80, 1975.

[9] Southward K. The Systemic Theory of Dental Caries. Gen Dent 59(5): 367-73, 2011.

[10] Leonora J, Tieche J-M, Steinman RR. The Effect of Dietary Factors on Intradentinal Dye Penetration in the Rat. Archs oral Biol 37(9):733-41, 1992.

[11] Steinman RR. Pharmacologic Control of Dentinal Fluid Movement and Dental Caries in Rats. J Dent Res 47(5): 720-24, 1968.

[12] Steinman RR, Leonora J. Physiologic resistance to dental caries. J Missouri Dent Assn 57(3): 14-21, 1977.

[13] Leonora J, Tieche J-M, Steinman RR. Further evidence for a hypothalamus-parotid gland endocrine axis in the rat. Arch Oral Biol 38: 911-16, 1993.

[14] Tieche J-M, Leonora J, Steinman RR. High-sucrose diet inhibits basal secretion of intradentinal dye penetration-stimulating parotid hormone in pigs. J Appl Physiol 76: 218-22, 1994.

[15] Steinman RR, Leonora J. *Dentinal Fluid Transport*. (Loma Linda, California: The Loma Linda University Press, 2004), xv.

[16] Ciucchi B, Bouillaquet S, Holz J, et al. Dentinal fluid dynamics in human teeth, in vivo. J Endod 21(4): 191-4, 1995.

[17] Fish EW. The circulation of lymph in dentin and enamel. J Am dent Ass 14: 804-17, 1927.

[18] Bodeck CF, Lefkowitz W. Concerning the "vitality" of the calcified dental tissues. J Dent Res 16: 463-75, 1937.

[19] Berggren H. Penetration of dyes in living human enamel. J Dent Res 22: 1-6, 1943.

[20] von Kreudenstein S. Uber den Dentinloquor. Schweiz med Wschr 88: 635-39, 1958.

[21] von Kreudenstein S. Contributions to the biochemistry of dental lymph. New York State Dent J 24:343-47, 1958.

[22] Potts TV, Cunningham T, Finkelstein MJ, et al. Arch Oral Biol 30(4): 353-7, 1985.

[23] Litovsky B, Arancibia S. Modification by ouabaine et colchicine du flux transdentinaire estime in vivo par perfusion: "push-pull" d'incisives de rat. J Biol buccale 16: 209-14, 1988.

[24] Lefkowitz W. Further observations of dental lymph in the dentin. J Dent Res 22: 287-92, 1943.

[25] Sognnaes RF, Shaw JH, Bogoroch R. Radiotracer studies on bone, cementum, dentin and enamel of rhesus monkeys. Am J Physiol 180(2): 408-20, 1955.

[26] Pashley DH, Nelson R, Pashley EL. In vivo fluid movement across dentine in the dog. Archs Oral Biol 26:707-10, 1981.

[27] Pashley DH, Kehl T, Pashley E, et al. Comparison of in vitro and in vivo dog dentin permeability. J Dent Res 60: 763-8, 1981.

[28] Leonora J, Steinman RR. Evidence suggesting the existence of a hypothalamic-parotid gland endocrine axis. Endocrinology 83: 807-15, 1968.

[29] Leonora J, Tieche J-M, Celestin J. Physiological factors affecting secretion of parotid hormone. Am J Physiol 252 (Endocrinol Metab): E477-84, 1987.

[30] Steinman RR, Leonora J. Suppression of dental caries by chemical activation of the hypothalamic-parotid endocrine axis. J Dent Res 48: S207, 1969.

[31] Leonora J, Steinman RR. Evidence suggesting the existence of a hypothalamic-parotid gland endocrine axis. Endocrinology 83: 807-15, 1968.

[32] Leonora J, Tieche J-M, Steinman RR. Further evidence for a hypothalamus-parotid gland endocrine axis in the rat. Arch Oral Biol 38: 911-16, 1993.

[33] Zhang Q, Szalay AA, Tieche J-M, et al. Cloning and functional study of porcine parotid hormone, a novel proline-rich protein. J Biol Chem 280(23): 22233-44, 2005.

[34] Nyvad B, ten Cate JM, Fejerskov O. Arrest of root surface caries in situ. J Dent Res 76: 1845-53, 1997.

[35] Steinman RR. The physiologic nature of caries susceptibility - Part III. J Alabama Dent Assn 67: 46-49, 1983.

[36] Steinman RR. The physiologic nature of caries susceptibility - Part III. J Alabama Dent Assn 67: 46-49, 1983.

# Chapter 10

[1] Steinman RR, Leonora J. Evidence suggesting the existence of a hypothalamic-parotid gland endocrine axis. Endocrinology 83:807-815, 1968.

[2] Steinman RR, Leonora J. Suppression of dental caries by chemical activation of the hypothalamic-parotid endocrine axis. J Dent Res 48:S207, Abstr #666, 1969.

[3] Steinman RR, Leonora J. Relationship of Fluid Transport Through the Dentin to the Incidence of Dental Caries. J Dent Res 50(6):1536-42, 1971.

[4] Steinman RR, Leonora J, Tieche J-M. Susceptibility to dental caries. Aust Dent J 24(4): 222-4, 1979.

[5] Leonora J, Tieche J-M, Steinman RR. Stimulation of Intradentinal Dye Penetration by Feeding in the Rat. Archs Oral Biol. 38(9):763-69, 1993.

[6] Steinman RR, Leonora J, Singh RJ. The effect of desalivation upon pulpal function and dental caries in rats. J Dent Res 59(2): 176-185, 1980.

[7] Steinman RR. Pharmacologic Control of Dentinal Fluid Movement and Dental Caries in Rats. J Dent Res 47(5):720-24, 1968.

[8] Steinman RR. The Movement of Acriflavine Hydrochloride Through Molars of Rats on a Cariogenic and Non-Cariogenic Diet. J South Calif Dent Assoc 35:151-7, 1967.

[9] Steinman RR. The Effect of Pyridoxine and Injected Carbohydrate on Incidence of Caries, Dentinal Circulation Related to Diet. J Dent Res 37: 874-79, 1958.

[10] Yagiela JA, Dowd FJ, Neidle EA. *Pharmacology and Therapeutics for Dentistry* 5th ed. (St. Louis: Mosby, Inc, 2004), 84-97.

[11] Beers MH, Fletcher AJ, Jones TV, et al. *The Merck Manual of Medical Information* 2nd ed. (Whitehouse Station: Merck Research Laboratories, 2003), 5, 437.

[12] Yagiela JA, Dowd FJ, Neidle EA. *Pharmacology and Therapeutics for Dentistry* 5th ed. (St. Louis: Mosby, Inc, 2004), 565.

[13] Palacios R, Sugawara I. Hydrocortisone abrogates proliferation of T cells in autologous mixed lymphocyte reaction by rendering the interleukin-2 Producer T cells unresponsive to interleukin-1 and unable to synthesize the T-cell growth factor. Scand Journal of Immunology 15(1): 25-31, 1982.

[14] Kucharz EJ. Hormonal control of collagen metabolism. Part II. Endocrinologie 26(4): 229-37, 1988.

[15] Nelson RF. *An Introduction to Behavioral Endocrinology* 4th ed. (Sunderland, Mass: Sinauer Associated Inc, 2011).

[16] Mustoe AC, Bimie AK, Korgan AC, et al. Natural variation in gestational cortisol is associated with patterns of growth in mamoset monkeys (Callithrix geoffroyi). Gen Comp Endocrinol 175(3): 519-26, 2012.

[17] Marucha PT, Kiecolt-Glaser JK, Favagehi M, et al. Mucosal wound healing is impaired by examination stress. Psychosom Med 60(3): 362-5, 1998.

[18] Liu FT, Lin HS Effect of Hydrocortisone Acetate on Dental Caries and Salivary Glands in Adrenalectomized Female Rats. J Dent Res 47(1):158-66, 1968.

[19] Besic FC, Zimmerman S, Normore W, et al. Caries Incidence in Cortisone-Treated Rats. J Dent Res 38: 687, 1959.

[20] Sweeney EA, Shaw JH. The Effect of Adrenalectomy and Cortisone Supplementation on Caries Incidence in Caries-Susceptible Rats. J Dent Res 44: 96-98, 1965.

[21] Ehrich WE, Seifter, J. Role Played by the Salivary Glands in the "Alarm Reaction." Arch Path 45: 239-245, 1948.

[22] Shafer WG, Muhler JC. The Relationship of the Salivary Glands, Endocrine System, and Dental Caries in the Albino Rats. J Dent Res 32: 684, 1953.

[23] Sutton PRN. Mental Stress and Acute Dental Caries. Nature 195: 254-256, 1962.

[24] Steinman RR, Smith LV. The effect of stress upon the incidence of dental caries. J South Calif Dent Assn 28(11): 367-9, 1960.

[25] Su N, Marek C, Ching V, et al. Caries Prevention for Patients with Dry Mouth. J Can Dent Assoc 77:b85, 2011.

[26] Roberson TM, Heymann HO, Swift EJ. *Sturdevant's Art & Science of Operative Dentistry*, 4th ed. (Chapel Hill, North Carolina: Mosby, Inc, 2002), 99.

[27] Bhathena SJ, Berlin E, Judd JT, et al. Effects of omega 3 fatty acids and vitamin E on hormones involved in carbohydrate and lipid metabolism in men. Am J Clin Nutr 54(4): 684-8, 1991.

[28] Delarue J, Matzinger O, Binnert C, et al. Fish oil prevents the adrenal activation elicited by mental stress in healthy men. Diabetes Metab 29(3): 289-95, 2003.

[29] Golf SW, Bender S, Gruttner J, et al. On the significance of magnesium in extreme physical stress. Cariovasc Drugs Ther 12 Suppl 2(2suppl): 197-202, 1998.

[30] Golf SW, Happel O, Graef V, et al. Plasma aldosterone, cortisol and electrolyte concentrations in physical exercise after magnesium supplementation. J Clin Chem Clin Biochem 22(11): 717-21, 1984.

[31] Dean C. *The Magnesium Miracle.*(New York: Ballantine Books, 2007), 230-33.

[32] Dean C. *The Magnesium Miracle.*(New York: Ballantine Books, 2007), 225.

[33] Field T, Hernandez-Reif M, Diego M, et al. Cortisol decreases and serotonin and dopamine increase following massage therapy. Int J Neurosci 115(10): 1397-413, 2005.

[34] Leproult R, Copinschi G, Buxton O, et al. Sleep loss results in an elevation of cortisol levels the next evening. Sleep 20(10): 865-70, 1997.

[35] Lovallo WR, Farag NH, Vincent AS, et al. Cortisol responses to mental stress, exercise, and meals following caffeine intake in men and women. Pharmacol Biochem Behav 83(3): 441-7, 2006.

[36] Berk LS, Tan SA, Berk D. Cortisol and Catecholamine stress hormone decrease is associated with the behavior of perceptual anticipation of mirthful laughter. The FASEB Journal 22(1): 946.11, 2008.

[37] Uedo N, Ishikawa H, Morimoto K, et al. Reduction in salivary cortisol level by music therapy during colonoscopic examination. Hepatogastroenterology 51(56): 451-3, 2004.

[38] Steinman R, Brussett M, Tartaryn P. Comparison of Caries Incidence in Exercised and Immobilized Rats. J Dent Res 40(1): 218, 1961.

[39] Quiroga MC, Bongard S, Kreutz G, et al. Emotional and Neurohumoral Responses to Dancing Tango Argentino: The Effects of Music and Partner. Music and Medicine 1(1): 14-21, 2009.

[40] Boyce WT, Den Besten PK, Stamperdahl J, et al. Social inequalities in childhood dental caries: the convergent roles of stress, bacteria and disadvantage. Soc Sci Med 71(9): 1644-52, 2010.

# Chapter 11

[1] Kronfeld R. *Histopathology of the Teeth and their Surrounding Structures*. (Philadelphia: Lea & Febiger,1939), 106.

[2] Leonora J, Tjaderhane L, Tieche JM. Parotid gland function and dentin apposition in rat molars. J Dent Res 81(4): 259-64, 2002.

[3] Howard BV, Wylie-Rosett J. AHA Scientific Statement. Circulation106: 523-527, 2002.

[4] "How to Spot Sugar on Food Labels," Permacology Productions Pty Ltd, assessed Feb 11, 2015, www.hungryforchange.tv/article/how-to-spot-sugar-on-food-labels.

[5] Casamassimo PS, Fields HW Jr, McTigue DJ, Nowak AJ. *Pediactric Dentistry Infancy through Adolescence* 4th ed. (St. Louis, Missouri: Elsevier Saunder, 2005), 320.

[6] "How to Spot Sugar on Food Labels," Permacology Productions Pty Ltd, assessed Feb 11, 2015,www.hungryforchange.tv/article/how-to-spot-sugar-on-food-labels.

[7] Steinman RR. The physiologic nature of caries susceptibility - Part III. J Alabama Dent Assn 67: 46-49, 1983.

[8] Cury JA, Rebelo MA, Del Bel Cury AAm et al. Biochemical composition and cariogenicity of dental plaque formed in the presence of sucrose or glucose or fructose. Caries Res. 2000; 34:491-7.

[9] "Vitamin Library: Molybdenum," DrWeil.com, accessed Feb 19, 2015, http://www.drweil.com/drw/u/ART03381/Molybdenum.html.

[10] "Supplements & Herbs: Zinc," DrWeil.com, accessed Feb 19, 2015, http://www.drweil.com/drw/u/ART02869/zinc.html.

[11] Steinman RR, Leonora J. Effect of selected dietary additives on the incidence of dental caries in the rat. J Dent Res 54(3): 570-77, 1975.

[12] "Supplements & Herbs: Zinc," DrWeil.com, accessed Feb 19, 2015, http://www.drweil.com/drw/u/ART02869/zinc.html.

[13] "Supplements & Herbs: Zinc," DrWeil.com, accessed Feb 19, 2015, http://www.drweil.com/drw/u/ART02869/zinc.html.

[14] Ballentine R. *Diet & Nutrition A Holistic Approach* (Honesdale, PA: Himalayan Institute Press, 2005), 239.

[15] "Supplements & Herbs: Chromium," DrWeil.com, accessed Feb 19, 2015, http://www.drweil.com/drw/u/ART02868/chromium.html.

[16] "Supplements & Herbs: Chromium," DrWeil.com, accessed Feb 19, 2015, http://www.drweil.com/drw/u/ART02868/chromium.html.

[17] Johnson S. The multifaceted and widespread pathology of magnesium deficiency. Med Hypotheses 56(2): 163-70, 2001.

[18] Southward K. The Systemic Theory of Dental Caries. Gen Dent 59(5): 367-73, 2011.

[19] Jauslin ML, Meier T, Smith RA, et al. Mitochondria-targeted antioxidants protect Friedreich Ataxia fibroblasts from endogenous oxidative stress more effectively than untargeted antioxidants. FASEB J 17(13): 1972-4, 2003.

[20] Packer L, Colman C. *The Antioxidant Miracle* (MA: John Wiley & Sons, Inc, 1999), 55, 78, 92, 106, 118.

[21] Alvares JO. Nutrition, tooth development, and dental caries. Am J Clin Nutr 61(2): 410S-416S,1995.

[22] "Hunger What is Malnutrition?" World Food Programme, assessed Feb 11, 2015, http://www.wfp.org/hunger/malnutrition.

[23] Roberson TM, Heymann HO, Swift EJ. *Sturdevant's Art & Science of Operative Dentistry*, 4th ed. (Chapel Hill, North Carolina: Mosby, Inc, 2002), 103.

[24] Steinman RR. The physiologic nature of caries susceptibility - Part III. J Alabama Dent Assn 67: 46-49, 1983.

[25] Larmas M, Dental Caries Seen from the Pulpal Side: a Non-traditional Approach. J Dent Res 82(4): 253-6, 2003.

[26] Kortelainen S, Larmas M. Effects of low and high fluoride levels on rate of dentin apposition and caries progression in young and old Wistar rats. Scand J Dent Res 102: 30-3, 1994.

[27] Stanley HR, Pereira JC, Spiegel E, et al. The detection and prevalence of reactive and physiologic sclerotic dentin, reparative dentin and dead tracts beneath various types of dental lesions according to tooth surface and age. J Oral Pathol 12(4): 257-89, 1983.

[28] Roberson TM, Heymann HO, Swift EJ. *Sturdevant's Art & Science of Operative Dentistry*, 4th ed. (Chapel Hill, North Carolina: Mosby, Inc, 2002), 146.

[29] Fried K. Changes in innervation of dentine and pulp with age. In Ferguson DF, editor: The aging mouth, Basel, 1987, Karger.

[30] Roberson TM, Heymann HO, Swift EJ. *Sturdevant's Art & Science of Operative Dentistry*, 4th ed. (Chapel Hill, North Carolina: Mosby, Inc, 2002), 146.

[31] Roberson TM, Heymann HO, Swift EJ. *Sturdevant's Art & Science of Operative Dentistry*, 4th ed. (Chapel Hill, North Carolina: Mosby, Inc, 2002), 148.

[32] Roberson TM, Heymann HO, Swift EJ. *Sturdevant's Art & Science of Operative Dentistry*, 4th ed. (Chapel Hill, North Carolina: Mosby, Inc, 2002), 148.

[33] Steinman RR. Can dental caries susceptibility be affected by the ingestion of carbohydrates? J Indiana State Dent Assoc 39: 130-4, Aprtil 1960.

[34] Leonora J, Tjaderhane L, Tieche JM. Parotid gland function and dentin apposition in rat molars. J Dent Res 81(4): 259-64, 2002.

[35] Tjaderhane L, Hietala EL, Larmas M. Reducation in dentine apposition in rat molars by a high-sucrose diet. Arch Oral Biol 39(6): 491-5, 1994.

[36] Steinman RR, Leonora J. *Dentinal Fluid Transport.* (Loma Linda, California: The Loma Linda University Press, 2004), 97- 101.

[37] Leonora J, Tjaderhane L, Tieche JM. Parotid gland function and dentin apposition in rat molars. J Dent Res 81(4): 259-64, 2002.

[38] Leonora J, Tjaderhane L, Tieche JM. Effect of dietary carbamyl phosphate on dentine apposition in rat molars. Arch Oral Biol 47: 147-53, 2002.

[39] Steinman RR, Leonora J. *Dentinal Fluid Transport.* (Loma Linda, California: The Loma Linda University Press, 2004), 97- 101.

[40] Roberson TM, Heymann HO, Swift EJ. *Sturdevant's Art & Science of Operative Dentistry,* 4th ed. (Chapel Hill, North Carolina: Mosby, Inc, 2002), 23.

[41] Roberson TM, Heymann HO, Swift EJ. *Sturdevant's Art & Science of Operative Dentistry,* 4th ed. (Chapel Hill, North Carolina: Mosby, Inc, 2002), 69.

[42] Julian D, Boyd MD, Drain CL. The Arrest of Dental Caries in Childhood. JAMA 90(23); 1867-9, 1928.

[43] Julain D, Boyd MD, Drain CL. Dietary Control of Dental Caries. *Am J Dis Child* 38(4): 721-5, 1929.

[44] Julain D, Boyd MD, Drain CL. Dietary Control of Dental Caries. *Am J Dis Child* 38(4): 721-5, 1929.

[45] Julain D, Boyd MD, Drain CL. Dietary Control of Dental Caries. *Am J Dis Child* 38(4): 721-5, 1929.

[46] Mellanby M, Coumoulos H. Improved Dentition of 5-year-old London School-children. Br Med J 1(4355): 837–840, 1944.

[47] Price WA. *Nutrition and Physical Degeneration* 8th ed. (La Mesa, CA: Price-Pottenger Nutrition Foundation, 2008),260-1.

[48] Holick MF. Resurrection of vitamin D deficiency and rickets. J Clin Invest 116(8):2062–72, 2006.

[49] Agnew MC, Agnew RG, Tisdall FF. The production and prevention of dental caries. J Pediatr 2(2): 190-211, 1933.

[50] Marshall CD, Sedwick HJ. The Fat-Soluble Vitamins and Dental Caries in Children. J Nutr 8(3): 309-28, 1934.

[51] McBeath EC. Experiments On the Dietary Control of Dental Caries in Children. J Dent Res12: 723-47, 1932.

[52] Anderson PG, Williams CHM, Halderson H, et al.The Influence of Vitamin D in the Prevention of Dental Caries. J Am Dent 21(8): 1349-66, 1934.

[53] McBeath EC, Zucker TF. The Role of Vitamin D in the Control of Dental Caries in Children. J Nutr 15(6): 547-64, 1938.

[54] Hujoel PP. Vitamin D and dental caries in controlled clinical trials: systematic review and meta-analysis. Nutrition Reviews 71(2): 88-97, 2013.

[55] Bonucci E, Lozupone E, Silvestrini G, et al. Morphological studies of hypomineralized enamel of rat pups on calcium-deficient diet, and of its changes after return to normal diet. Anat Rec 239(4): 379-95, 1994.

[56] Rude RK, Adams JS, Ryzen E, et al. Low serum concentrations of 1,25-dihydroxyvitamin D in human magnesium deficiency. J Clin Endocrinol Metab 61: 833-940, 1985.

[57] Dean C. *The Magnesium Miracle.*(New York: Ballantine Books, 2007), lxxvii.

[58] Dean C. *The Magnesium Miracle.*(New York: Ballantine Books, 2007), 20.

[59] Dean C. *The Magnesium Miracle.*(New York: Ballantine Books, 2007), 14.

[60] Tsuboi S, Nakagaki H, Ishiguro K, et al. Magnesium distribution in human bone. Calcif Tissue Int 54(1): 34-7, 1994.

[61] Steinfort J, Driessens FC, Heijligers HJ, et al. The distribution of magnesium in developing rat incisor dentin. J Dent Res 70(3): 187-91, 1991.

[62] Iseri LT, French JH. Magnesium: nature's physiologic calcium blocker. Am Heart J 108: 188-193, 1984.

[63] Seelig MS, "Cardiovascular reactions to stress intensified by magnesium deficit in consequences of magnesium deficiency on the enhancement of stress reactions: preventive and therapeutic implications: a review." J Am Coll Nutr, vol. 13, no. 5, pp, 429-446, 1994.

[64] Orban B. Nutrition and teeth. J Am Dent Assoc 14: 1619, 1927.

[65] Harris SS, Navia JM. Vitamin A deficiency and caries susceptibility of rat molars. Arch Oral Biol 25(6): 415-21, 1980.

[66] Scuster GS, Dirksen TR, Ciarlone AE, et al. Anticaries and antiplaque potential of free-fatty acids in vitro and in vivo. Pharmacol Ther Dent 5(1-2): 25-33, 1980.

[67] Bown WH. Food components and caries. Adv Dent Res 8(2): 215-20, 1994.

[68] Steinman RR. Can dental caries susceptibility be affected by the ingestion of carbohydrates? J Indiana State Dent Assoc 39: 130-4, April 1960.

[69] Erickson PR, Mazhari E. Investigation of the role of human breast milk in caries development. Pediatr Dent 21: 86, 1999.

[70] Casamassimo PS, Fields HW Jr, McTigue DJ, Nowak AJ. *Pediactric Dentistry Infancy through Adolescence* 4th ed. (St. Louis, Missouri: Elsevier Saunder, 2005), 204.

[71] Steinman RR. Can dental caries susceptibility be affected by the ingestion of carbohydrates? J Indiana State Dent Assoc 39: 130-4, April 1960.

[72] "Vitamin D Fact Sheet for Health Professionals," National Institutes of Health, accessed Feb 19, 2015, http://ods.od.nih.gov/factsheets/VitaminD-HealthProfessional/.

[73] Flore R, Ponziani FR, DiRienzo TA, et al. Something more to say about calcium homeostasis: the role of vitamin K2 in vascular calcification and osteoporosis. Eur Rev Med Pharmacol Sci 17: 2433-40, 2013.

[74] Hegde MN, Kumari S, Hegde ND, et al. Relation Between Salivary and Serum Vitamin C Levels and Dental Caries Experience in Adults – A Biochemical Study. Nitte University Journal of Health Science 3(4): 2013.

# Chapter 12

[1] "National Oral Health Call to Action," Carmona RH, Acting Assistant Secretary for Health United States Surgeon General U.S. Department of Health and Human Services, 2003, assessed Feb 16, 2015, http://www.surgeongeneral.gov/news/speeches/oralhealth042903.html.

[2] Kidd EAM, Fejerskov O. What Constitutes Dental Caries? Histopathology of Carious Enamel and Dentin Related to the Action of Cariogenic Biofilms. J Dent Res 83(Spec Iss C): C35-C38, 2004.

[3] Roberson TM, Heymann HO, Swift EJ. *Sturdevant's Art & Science of Operative Dentistry*, 4th ed. (Chapel Hill, North Carolina: Mosby, Inc, 2002), 109.

[4] Roberson TM, Heymann HO, Swift EJ. *Sturdevant's Art & Science of Operative Dentistry*, 4th ed. (Chapel Hill, North Carolina: Mosby, Inc, 2002), 108.

[5] Roberson TM, Heymann HO, Swift EJ. *Sturdevant's Art & Science of Operative Dentistry*, 4th ed. (Chapel Hill, North Carolina: Mosby, Inc, 2002), 109.

[6] Roberson TM, Heymann HO, Swift EJ. *Sturdevant's Art & Science of Operative Dentistry*, 4th ed. (Chapel Hill, North Carolina: Mosby, Inc, 2002), 109.

[7] Holmen L, Thylstrup A, Artun J. Clinical and histological features observed during arrestment of active enamel carious lesions in vivo. Caries Res 21: 546-54, 1987.

[8] Holmen L, Thylstrup A, Artun J. Surface changes during the arrest of active enamel carious lesions in vivo. A scanning electron microscopic study. Acta Odontol Scand 45: 383-390, 1987.

[9] Soderholm K-J M. Reactor paper. The impact of recent changes in the epidemiology of dental caries on guidelines for the use of dental sealants: clinical perspectives. J Public Health Dent 55:302, 1995.

[10] Casamassimo PS, Fields HW Jr, McTigue DJ, Nowak AJ. *Pediactric Dentistry Infancy through Adolescence* 4th ed. (St. Louis, Missouri: Elsevier Saunder, 2005), 531.

[11] Workshop on Guidelines for Sealant Use: Recommendations. J Public Health Dent 55:263, 1995.

[12] Ekstrand KR, Qvist V, Thylstrup A. Light microscope study of the effect of probing in occlusal surfaces. Caries Res 21: 368-74, 1987.

[13] Roberson TM, Heymann HO, Swift EJ. *Sturdevant's Art & Science of Operative Dentistry*, 4th ed. (Chapel Hill, North Carolina: Mosby, Inc, 2002), 408.

[14] Roberson TM, Heymann HO, Swift EJ. *Sturdevant's Art & Science of Operative Dentistry*, 4th ed. (Chapel Hill, North Carolina: Mosby, Inc, 2002), 97.

[15] Roberson TM, Heymann HO, Swift EJ. *Sturdevant's Art & Science of Operative Dentistry*, 4th ed. (Chapel Hill, North Carolina: Mosby, Inc, 2002), 102.

[16] Artun J, Thylstrup A. A three-year clinical and SEM study of surface changes of carious enamel lesions after inactivation. Am J Dentofac Orthop 95: 27-33, 1989.

[17] Roberson TM, Heymann HO, Swift EJ. *Sturdevant's Art & Science of Operative Dentistry*, 4th ed. (Chapel Hill, North Carolina: Mosby, Inc, 2002), 103.

[18] Kidd EAM, Fejerskov O. What Constitutes Dental Caries? Histopathology of Carious Enamel and Dentin Related to the Action of Cariogenic Biofilms. J Dent Res 83(Spec Iss C): C35-C38, 2004.

[19] Roberson TM, Heymann HO, Swift EJ. *Sturdevant's Art & Science of Operative Dentistry*, 4th ed. (Chapel Hill, North Carolina: Mosby, Inc, 2002), 408.

# Index

MMPs and, *113*
nutrition and, *189*
remineralization likeliness
    chart, *32*
remineralization of, 213
dextromaltose, *193*
digestion, 74, 97, 163, *186, 205*
distilled water, *103*
dye penetration, *155*

# E

eburnated dentin, *21, 22, 218,
    219*
eggs, *196, 197, 199*
eggshells, *187*
emotions, *164, 173, 186*
enzymes, 97
epinephrine. *See* adrenaline
esophageal receptors, 98
estrogen
    breast cancer and, *148*
    cavities and, 143
    metabolism, *145–47*
    odontoblasts and, 143
exercise
    and cavities, 171
    damage due to excessive, 125
    damaging effects of excessive,
        186
    estrogen decreasing, 146
    stress reduction and, 171
explorer, 215, 219, 224
    damage caused by, 215
    for tartar detection, 217
    in between teeth, 217

# F

Facebook, *176*
failure to thrive, 12
fatigue, 63

feed supplement. *See* ammonium
    chloride
fermented food, 87, 206
fertility, *165*
fibroblasts, *150*
fight or flight response, *163, 164*
fillings
    amalgam, 8
    bisphenol A (BPA), 8
    composite, 8
    longevity, 7
    mercury, 8
    recurrent decay, 7
fish, *184*
flaking enamel, 28
flame retardant, 140
flavonoid, 81
flax seeds, *169*
fluoride, 5, *158, 195*
food
    cooked starches, 105
    raw, 105
    saliva and, 105
food additive (E510). *See*
    ammonium chloride
free radicals
    naked molecules analogy, 120
fruit, *196, 197, 201*

# G

GAPS, 89
genetics, *49, 73, 195*
glucose, *205*
    dentin fluid and, 179
    in sucrose, 178
    injected, 154
    measuring in blood, 178
    tooth susceptibility and, 179
glucosinolate glucobrassicin, 146
glycemic index, *180*
goldenseal, 82
Gram-positive bacteria, *204*

magnesium deficiency and,
125
redox signaling, 122
tests, 127
oxygen radical absorbance
capacity. *See* ORAC

## P

pain, 11, 214, 220
parasympathetic nervous system,
*164*
cavities and, 166
parotid hormone and, 167
parathyroid hormone, 134, 202
parotid gland, 155, 162, 163,
262, 263, 264
parotid hormone
and eating, *159*
animal research and, *154*
as protection, *159*
discovery of, *154*
DNA sequencing of, *157*
dye penetration of, *155*
effect on dentin fluid, *156*
future supplementation of,
*157*
hypothalamus and, *157*
pecans, *170*
perimenopause, *145*
periodontal disease. *See* gum
disease
Periostat, 117
Peru, *189*
pesticide, 125, 140, 147
pH, 51–75
how to test, 58
infants and children, 58
measurement of acid, 52
schedule for testing, 59
'the critical pH', 55
pH paper, 57

phosphate, 53, 54, 55, 97, 104,
187, 205, 270
phthalates, 147
proanthocyanidin, 126
probiotics, 87–89
professional cleanings
arrested decay and, 222
progesterone, *145*
proximal surface. *See*
interproximal surface
pulp, *150*, *153*
adult pulp chambers, *192*
blood supply and
remineralization, *168*
capping, *23*
cavities extending into, *38*
clove and, *81*
components of, *150*
function of, *150*
location, *19*
odontoblasts and, *20*, *21*
pumpkin seeds, *169*
puzzle pieces analogy, 25

## R

radioactive fluids, 154
Ralph Steinman, *160*
recurrent decay, 7, 30
as superficial staining, 32
in remineralization likeliness
chart, 32
red wine, 222
redox signaling, 122
relapse. *See* orthodontics
remineralization
as an option in the modern
dental office, 212
as prevention, 10
color changes and, 221
developing teeth, 213
doesn't matter what technique
is used, 229

early experiments of, 196
explorer damage and, 215
function of saliva, 97
gift for children, 194
how long it takes, *39, 197*
more effort needed, 6
natural approaches to, 5
seeing a dentist for, 210
unsuccessful, 212
vitamin D and, *203*
remineralization likeliness chart,
*31–35*
resting saliva. *See* unstimulated
saliva
rickets, *202*

# S

saliva
food and, 105
medications and, 104
natural strategies to increase,
102
protective functions, 97
smoking and, 104
stimulated, 98
testing for water content, 99
unstimulated, 98
salivary gland
parotid. *See* parotid gland
submandibular, 143
salivary glands
bromine and, 138
depleted, 101
iodine receptors, 136
salt, *170*
school performance, 12, *202*
sclerotic dentin, *21, 22, 218, 219*
selenium, 119
skin wound analogy, 23
sleep, *170*
smoking, 104, 124
smooth surfaces, 26

sodium-iodide symporter, 136
*Steptococcus mutans, 204*
stevia, *182*
stimulated saliva, 98
testing for, 100
stomping on dirt analogy, 27
*Strepococcus mutans*
as MS bacteria, 78
*Streptococcus ferus*, 78
Streptococcus mutans. *See* MS
bacteria
*Streptococcus rattus*, 78
*Streptococcus sangria*, 78
stress
autonomic nervous system,
164
cavities and, 166–68
children experiencing, 172
cortisol, 165–66
dental students study, 166
free radical source, 125
missing puzzle piece to cavity
cause, 173
pH and, 66
saliva and, 104
self-hypnosis, 172
stress response, *163, 164*
submandibular salivary gland,
143, 240, 254, 255
sucrose, *178, 195, 205*
also known as, *180*
at mealtime, *182*
blood glucose and, *179*
composition of, *178*
dentin fluid effects on, *178*
increased susceptibility, *178*
sugar. *See* sucrose
supplements, *170*
antioxidants, 126
carbamoyl phosphate, 187
goldenseal, 82
indol-3-carbinol, 146
iodine, 138

maca, 147
magnesium, 170
minerals, 69
parotid hormone, 158
probiotics, 88
sympathetic nervous system, *163*
  cavities and, 166

# T

target cells, 132, 133, 136, 143,
  148
tea, *81*, *119*
teeth
  anatomy, 18–22
  can heal, 2
  cementum, 19
  crown, 19, 28
  crumbling, 29
  dentin, 19
  enamel, 19
  enamel thickness, 19
  hydroxyapatite, 19
  meant to remineralize, 6
  pulp, 19
  root, 19
testosterone, *145*
TIMP, 109
tissue inhibitor
  metalloproteinase. *See* TIMP
tomato juice, *197*
Tomes fibers, *20*, *150*
Type 2 diabetes, *180*

# U

unstimulated saliva, 98
  testing for, 99

# V

vaccine, *158*
vegetables, *183*, *196*, *197*

vitamin A, *199*, 203
vitamin C, 207
vitamin D, 202
  breast feeding and deficiency
    of, 206
vitamin D2, *199*
vitamin K$_2$, 206

# W

walnuts, *169*, *170*
water
  bicarbonate, 74
  chlorophyll drops, 68
  filters, 103
  lemon, 60, 72
  liquid minerals in, 69
  natural spring, 74
  OH + H, 54
  scalding vs ice analogy for
    acidity, 61
whole grains, *183*, *184*

# X

xenobiotics, 125
xenoestrogens, 147
X-rays
  alternatives to, 218, 220
  arrested decay and, 218
  monitoring decay, 217
  radiopaque, 218
  scar from arrested decay, 218
xylitol, 82, 243

# Z

zinc, *184*
ZOE, 81

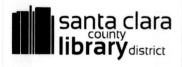